EAT THE YOLKS

YOLKS

discover Paleo, fight food lies, and reclaim your health

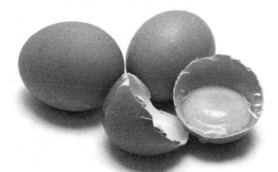

LIZ WOLFE, NTP

Victory Belt Publishing, Inc.
Las Vegas

For Spence.

Here's to a lifetime of adventures.

contents

foreword

At some point in our nutrition-and-health improvement journeys, which I presume you are on simply by the fact that you've picked up this book, we've likely figured out that we were misled or misguided somewhere along the way. Make no mistake about it, I too fell victim to the hype. You know what I'm talking about here, right? I'm talking about the "eating fat will make you fat" / "you need eleven servings of heart-healthy whole grains daily" / "anything made from soy is a health food" hype. If you didn't know that was hype before, you will now.

I was right there with you for many years, chowing down cereal made of seven whole grains on a mission (to kill you) with soy milk (it must be healthy, right?!), fat-free yogurt (sweetened with aspartame), nonstick cooking sprays (but they're low-fat!), and calorie-free sweeteners (that were "naturally" sweet). That is, until I saw the light.

For each of us, that "light" comes in a different form. If that light hasn't already been turned on for you, then you're in for a real treat. This book—and Liz's take on nutrition in general—will be that for you. And if that's the case, I am *stoked* for you. You are going to get your world flipped upside down and sideways while you learn exactly what is true about the food you eat every day. And you'll probably be smacking yourself upside the head when you realize that you've been fighting your instincts on what's right and wrong about nutrition, but you will definitely be ready to stop the diet-food-and-calorie-cutting madness.

This book will set you free from the 100-calorie-pack-filled world of edible foodlike substances that cry "healthy" on the package but are slowly making you sicker and sicker as you eat them. Yes, it's *that* dramatic. The impact that food has on your health is *that* serious. It's a good thing Liz, a Nutritional Therapy Practitioner (NTP™) certified by the Nutritional Therapy Association, has a seriously hilarious way of explaining it all.

Allow me to back up for just a moment, because I haven't known Liz my entire life, contrary to what our podcasting banter may imply. I was introduced to Liz Wolfe when listening to a podcast that was part of a (short-lived) series created by Hayley and Bill Staley (of *The Food Lovers Kitchen* and *Make It Paleo* fame) called "The Food Lovers Dish It." Liz was the featured guest on one of the episodes they recorded—and right away, I loved her voice.

Now, when I say that I loved Liz's voice, I mean both her audible voice *and* her way of thinking and presenting her opinions. I should tell you that I was feverishly on the hunt for a podcasting partner at this exact moment, so much so that I pulled my car over while driving on a busy highway to shoot Hayley a text and ask for Liz's contact information. That was the beginning of the end, some might say—and I mean that in the absolute *best* way possible.

That was several years ago now, and I've since not only convinced Liz to record a weekly podcast with me (the "Balanced Bites" podcast, which ranks in the top Health shows in iTunes), but also (literally) dragged her on the road with me to meet folks across the country and teach them why "everything you know about good nutrition is wrong"—and, of course, exactly how to get it right.

Through the development of the podcast and our seminar curriculum, I have seen deeper into Liz's passion and vigor for the Truth About Food (which could easily have been the title for this book, but that doesn't pack the same vitamin D–rich punch as *Eat the Yolks*). She wants to know more than just the biochemistry of nutrition; she wants to know the social and historical implications of the changes in our food supply—and what those changes have done to our long-term health.

Liz has a real knack for connecting with her readers (and our listeners and workshop attendees) in a way that is unlike anyone I've ever met. She isn't just hilarious; she is also darned *smart* about nutrition. Her passion for all things myth-and-truth-related when it comes to, oh, let's say the history of how the heck we started eating margarine, for example, has driven her to tirelessly research the foundations of it all. And she's able to turn around and tell you the story and actually make it interesting—injecting it with her signature wit and sense of humor—so that you leave the room never wanting to eat margarine again (and likely slapping it out of your spouse's or sibling's hand, too!).

In *Eat the Yolks,* Liz takes us step by step through nearly every dogmatic, scientifically unsound, and anti–"real food" notion that so many of us have been hung up on for years. She sheds light on the errors of those well-intentioned ways with compassion (she's been there too, folks) and wit. Liz explains why we need to eat fat (including saturated fat!), cholesterol, and even salt. (Bacon, yes! Steak, yes! Egg yolks, oh heck yes!)

Perhaps you've been bored to tears in the past by long, epic tomes that aim to educate you on the political and nutritional mess of what we've been told to eat for the last several decades. Or maybe you've read some real-food-centered books, but they were filled with overly science-y jargon or a rigid approach or way of eating that didn't leave you feeling empowered—or you quit reading partway through because you were flat-out bored. Well this, my friends, is the book for you.

Pour yourself a tall glass of home-brewed kombucha, whip up a nice frittata, and get ready to be edu-tained from cover to cover. And, for the sake of all that is decent in this world, you had better eat those yolks!

Diane Sanfilippo, BS, NC
Certified Nutrition Consultant and *New York Times*
bestselling author of *Practical Paleo* and *The 21-Day Sugar Detox*

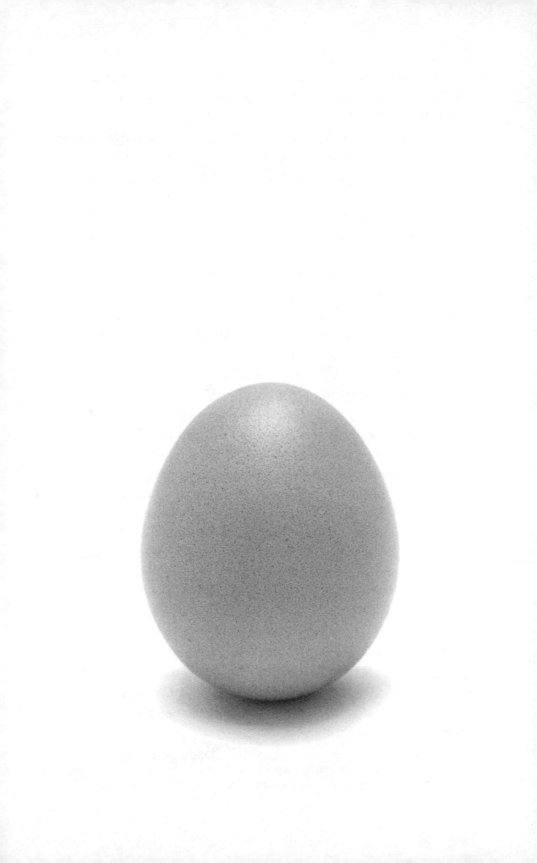

introduction

Happiness lies, first of all, in health.

GEORGE WILLIAM CURTIS

....

I wrote this book with the hope that we will soon see the last of the egg white omelet.

Truth time: We don't throw away egg yolks because we appreciate the culinary delight that is a rubbery, floppy, watery egg white breakfast. We do it because tossing that buttery, yellow-orange orb represents most of the ground rules of modern-day, so-called healthy eating: The cholesterol in egg yolks is bad for the heart. The calories in egg yolks can cause weight gain. The fat in egg yolks—well, a moment on the lips means a lifetime on the hips. Right?

The doctrine of modern nutrition proclaims that anything rich in cholesterol, calories, or saturated fat must be dangerous. Many even say that *all* animal products are unhealthy while all plant products are wholesome. Low-fat, low-carb, and low-calorie diets are all the rage, sometimes individually and sometimes all at once (oh, the hunger). If we believe the hype, the path to a better life is paved with the foods of conventional wisdom, our government's dietary recommendations, strict diet regimens, and sometimes in highly processed, packaged garbage marketed as "health food." And it's absolutely not paved with saturated fat, cholesterol, animal protein, carbs, or even salt. Because those things are bad, right?

Wrong.

Each and every one of those twisted takes on the truth has made victims of our bodies, our sanity, and our taste buds. The consequences of this nutrition dogma are visible everywhere: Rampant heart disease and obesity are major public health threats. Diet books are bestsellers year-round. Many people can't lose weight, and many others can't figure out why they feel just plain crappy when they're "doing everything right." Worse yet, many people haven't had a good steak in years out of fear for their health. That's a damn tragedy.

It's because everything we've been taught about good nutrition is wrong.

What if the foods we've been told not to eat—the foods we've been told might, in fact, kill us, make us fat, or make us unhealthy—are actually the foods we should be eating? What if the foods we've been told *are* healthy are actually causing us harm?

The only thing more infuriating than finding out that we've been lied to is finding out that we've been eating those lies for breakfast, lunch, and dinner, day in and day out, for decades. How could this have happened?

Here's the thing: From the time we're young, we place far more faith in so-called authorities than we do in our own common sense. This would make sense if we were talking brain surgery, but when it comes to eating—a basic, primal act that we are programmed to do, instinctively, from birth— it's simply outsourcing something that, deep down, we already know how to do. Unfortunately, we tend to accept what we're told, whether by a commercial, a label claim, or a so-called professional, rather than trusting what our instincts tell us. We grow up believing the lies, and they become the truths we live every day.

We don't always realize that the so-called authorities who spoon-feed us conventional wisdom about nutrition have been educated by corporate interests—or barely educated at all. Doctors, for example, don't get more than a few credit hours (if that) of nutritional education, and many nutrition professionals receive an education that is simply a regurgitation of the same old lies that this book is here to combat. Even dietitians are forced to endure a corporate-sponsored education: The Academy of Nutrition and Dietetics (formerly the American Dietetic Association), which is the credentialing body for all registered dietitians and associated educational programs in the United States, lists Coca-Cola, General Mills, Kellogg Company, SOYJOY, and other large processed-food conglomerates as major donors. (Of course, there are nutrition professionals who break the corporate mold, and every single one has my deepest gratitude.) But all too often, we listen not even to doctors and dietitians but to a plethora of pop experts proffering whatever fake-food-based diet catches on, whichever plan a celebrity swears by, or whatever obsessive, calorie-restrictive diet turned the Biggest Loser into the Smallest Winner—at least, until that Biggest Loser became the Biggest Regainer. We have to wonder: What the heck are we thinking?

The propaganda police (or how I learned to stop worrying and love real food)

I didn't think I was buying into the conventional nutritional wisdom until I asked myself a few questions. Take a moment, if you will, to answer them as well. Have you ever:

- Counted calories, points, or carbs?
- Stopped eating meat because you believed animal products were bad for you?

- Eaten soy-based meat or milk substitutes?
- Bought food that came in a box, bag, or package?
- Eaten something because it was labeled "fat-free"?
- Thrown away an egg yolk?
- Eaten margarine instead of butter?

If you answered "yes" to *any* of those questions, you're reading the right book.

If you answered "no" to those questions, you're probably *still* reading the right book. Because—even though I love you—I kinda think you're fibbing.

My passion for uncovering all the lies, where they came from, and why we believed them—and for writing this book—is rooted in my own transformation. Years ago, at the tail end of ten years of dieting disasters and robotlike adherence to deeply ingrained nutrition dogma, I was, yet again, feeling like a failure. I had tried everything, and not all of it with health in mind: I'd tried the ol' Red Bull–and–cigarettes diet and a few other desperate regimens in an attempt to eat less and drop the weight I'd gained on my college diet of beer and pizza. I dabbled in veganism, and, just to be contrarian, I followed that up with the Atkins diet. I did the lentil-soup-and-imitation-soy-cheese diet in an attempt to change my body (I spent most of that month sleeping). I tried eating "everything in moderation," counting calories based on my basal metabolic rate, counting points, and cutting carbs. I tried following the U.S. government's recommendations. And after ten years of this, I was confronted by the fact that I still wasn't healthy or happy, and that my relationship with food was totally deranged.

I was ready for a change, but I had no clue where to start. In fact, it hit me like a ton of bricks: I had no idea how to make my own life better. I'd failed miserably so many times, and I was afraid that history would repeat itself yet again.

Desperate, I enlisted the help of legendary strength and conditioning coach Michael Rutherford. I hoped "Coach Rut" would help me exercise my frustration away. Maybe he'd recommend a good protein shake or help me find a way to cut more calories without passing out on the way to the break room for my fifth cup of coffee.

What happened next was a turning point.

Coach Rut wasn't only dedicated to strength and conditioning. He was also dedicated to real food. He wasn't peddling low-fat dogma, protein bars, or calorie restriction. His philosophy was simple: If you want to feel better, you've got to eat better. That was when the magic would happen. I came for a workout (and a workout I got) and left with a much-needed reality check. It was time to change what I chose to eat and how I thought about food.

I knew Coach Rut was a fan of something called "Paleo." On this crazy (I thought) plan, you ate like a modern hunter-gatherer. This meant you ditched everything out of a box or a bag—even bread and pasta—and anything with a long list of unpronounceable ingredients. You ate only foods you could wrangle, if you had to, with your own hands: properly raised animals, vegetables, nuts, and fruits. You ate the *whole egg*. And steak. And avocado, in all its fatty glory. And a whole range of foods I'd long relegated to the nutrition boneyard like toys with broken squeakers.

Up until then, I'd always thought of food as an enemy. I only knew rules, "yes/no" lists, and the holy terror of calorie-counting paired with backslides of binge eating. I knew how to cry over a gallon of low-fat ice cream while watching *The Biggest Loser* and then eat high-fiber cereal with almond milk the next day to atone for my failings. I knew how to follow a vegan diet, a low-carb diet, or a low-fat diet as a clever disguise for cutting extreme amounts of calories. I knew how to be "on the wagon" and I knew how to be "off the wagon," but I didn't know how to live happily and healthfully without all that diet drama. I thought I was supposed to have willpower, but it seemed to fail me every time.

I asked myself: *Am I healthier for all the dietary insanity? Did all the wasted egg yolks, the diet food, and the conventional wisdom translate to a healthier, happier life?* My answer was, of course, no.

So I went Paleo, full-tilt. And something incredible happened.

I got healthier and happier simply by following a Paleo plan. My skin became clearer. My energy level was consistently high, and I slept well, waking up refreshed for the first time in years. I loved my life and my body. Turns out, it wasn't about willpower. It was about eating some emotion-balancing, hunger-regulating, body-nourishing real food and, above all, learning what junk was—and eliminating it.

Yet while I was thrilled with these changes, I still had lingering fears. I was worried that one day, I'd suddenly blow up like Violet Beauregarde in *Charlie and the Chocolate Factory* thanks to all the delicious, filling fat I was eating. I worried that the cholesterol in my egg yolks would give me heart disease. I worried that forgoing bread would somehow make me fiber-deficient and my—ahem—*regularity* was doomed to suffer. When I told people I was "eating Paleo," I didn't have a good answer when the inevitable questions came flooding in: *Won't all that animal protein give you cancer? Aren't you worried about your cholesterol? Is it really smart to eliminate all grains?* (Ironically, nobody seemed to care when my breakfast, lunch, and dinner consisted of nicotine and caffeine-laden soft drinks.)

For the first time, I wasn't content with simply following rules. I wanted to know why this was working and whether all the worries were justified. I wanted to know everything. With no dog in the fight, I set out to discover the truth about food, nutrition, and how I could best nourish my body. I wanted to know how we got here, why we believe what we believe, and what all of it meant to my health.

I read. I researched. I accumulated credentials in the worlds of both fitness and food: I received my CrossFit Level 1 trainer certificate and, soon after, I became a Nutritional Therapy Practitioner (NTP™) certified by the Nutritional Therapy Association. I began working toward my master's degree in public health so that I could better grasp the scope and the legitimacy of the research behind different ways of eating and better understand the shocking disease statistics that we've seen since certain foods fell out of favor. I started working with clients both individual and corporate, co-hosting a podcast, and traveling across the country to teach the principles of healthy eating to thousands of others. Over time, my interests shifted toward sustainable agriculture and self-sufficiency, so along with my incredible husband, I moved to a fifteen-acre homestead in the Midwest to start raising and growing our own food—the same foods I've been eating this whole time, only now they're homegrown. All the while, I've been documenting my personal journey on—you guessed it—a blog. (Because you're nobody until you're putting your every thought on the Internet.)

In my years of hacking away at nutrition lies and dusting the cobwebs off the truth, here is what I've discovered:

- We're told to choose foods based on myths that have absolutely no place in our dietary decision-making. Many of these myths are simply silly superstitions. Others are downright dangerous.

- The history behind the demonization of cholesterol, saturated fat, and animal products is quite shocking and has no nutritional validity. For the last sixty years, we have been the subjects of a nutrition experiment, and it has not gone well: We're more confused and less healthy than ever.

- Low-carb, low-fat, and low-calorie diets aren't all they're cracked up to be. It's the nutrient value and the quality of our food that matter most.

- Much of what we're told to eat is neither nutritious nor natural. It's processed junk disguised as health food, and it has the muscle of powerful industries behind it.

- When we strip away all the processing, the profitable industry, the diet dogma, and the bad science, we're left only with real food.

That last one is the most important point of all. When we're left with real food, we're left with the food that has a long history in the human diet. This is the food that humans—our ancestors—ate for thousands of years in good health, without fear.

Thanks to some of the better endeavors of nutritional science, we can look more closely at these real foods for insight into which nutrients we need most. This goes beyond just a Paleo diet to truly explore nutrients, where they come from, and why we need them.

Eating real, natural foods with a long history in the human diet isn't hard. Unlearning all the crap we've been taught? *That's* hard.

Before we get to all that, however, it's time to define some terms: what *Paleo, real food, and properly raised* really mean.

What we talk about when we talk about Paleo

Paleo is not a diet. It's not a fad. It's not a rigid set of rules to follow. It's not a sound bite. It's an exploration of history, nutrition, the human diet, and, most important, our health.

Paleo is the word we use to encompass a robust collection of information that continues to grow. This is not something that's been seen before in the "diet world," where lists of rules trump all and conventional wisdom, along with obsessive behavior, continues to reign.

Paleo is a term that helps define real food, the food with a long history in the human diet. It's the food our ancestors instinctively knew provided the greatest nutrition, and the food our modern knowledge of nutrition can verify as the most nutrient-dense. It's the only food that has *always* been food in some form: meat, eggs, and fat from healthy, properly raised animals and seafood; vegetables and fruits of all kinds; and a few lesser-known foods that we'll discuss in chapter 4.

Paleo is about learning from our ancestors and adopting modern versions of the behaviors that kept them healthy. And when I talk about our ancestors, I'm not just talking about cavemen and -women. I'm also talking about more recent hunter-gatherer cultures and isolated communities (often called "traditional cultures") that had no access to modern, processed foods and that lived off the natural resources available to them in great health, suffering none of the chronic diseases of our modern world. To guide our modern dietary decisions, we can search for common threads among what these cultures ate, the nutrition they valued, and how they thrived. Some of the foods they ate might seem surprising, like those discussed in chapter 4. Other foods are to be expected: meat and fat from properly raised animals, seafood, eggs, vegetables, fruits, and nuts. These are all *real foods,* and this book will explain that concept further. In talking about the shady, shocking history behind the demonization of these foods in our modern world, we will also be able to answer the question: *How the heck did we get to where we are today?*

Most important, eating well and healthfully means knowing where your food comes from. Throughout this book, we'll discuss "properly raised" animals and the importance of eating foods produced in a natural, harmonious environment. Factory farming, like much of industrial agriculture, is unnatural and inexcusable. Animals should be raised on their natural diets, in their natural environments, with the freedom to engage in their natural behaviors. That's what *properly raised* means—cattle graze on grass in open pasture instead of being fed corn on a feedlot; chickens range freely over pasture and eat insects, grass, and worms. A healthy animal makes healthy food, and this concept is vital to eating and living well. We are what our animals ate, after all. Fortunately, the Paleo movement has been—and continues to be—instrumental in making real, nutritious, properly raised animal products more accessible and more affordable.

Sound good? It should!

Before we move on, let's talk for a moment about the most pervasive propaganda that, at times, paralyzes us and makes us question our choices. Even the most commonsense concepts are often saddled with controversy, and Paleo is no exception. I want you to be prepared for the various things people may say to bomb your bacon.

But that's not *Paleo*

Remember, we're making choices based on a framework we call *Paleo,* and that's an entirely different animal from a list of rules defining so-called Paleo and non-Paleo foods. While it's tempting to make a rigid list, here's the problem: *Nothing* is Paleo if we go by black-and-white logic.

After all, almost all modern foods, including meat, vegetables, fruits, and nuts, were unavailable to our hunter-gatherer ancestors. The modern grass-fed Jersey cow has been around for just a few hundred years, and the modern beefsteak tomato was certainly not growing in lovely cave gardens. Fruit has been selectively bred over hundreds of years for maximum sweetness and size, while the fruit available thousands of years ago was small, tart, and a rare find.

Whatever cavemen could find, they'd probably eat—they had to survive, after all. We modern humans, however, have the luxury of abundant food. We just need guidelines to help us make wise choices.

The word *Paleo* simply represents the foods eaten before feedlots, global commerce, the refinement of sugar and grains, and the hydrogenation of fats changed our food landscape from one of nutritious, natural food to one of easy, cheap, and shelf-stable products. It represents a time when real fat was cherished as the nutrient-rich, nourishing food it is, when egg yolks were never thrown away, and when we weren't so damn confused by nutrition dogma that we completely lost our ability to recognize real food. It represents a time when heart disease, diabetes, autoimmunity, and diet-peddling TV doctors were virtually unknown.

So if you're concerned as to whether a steaming-hot, buttered potato is "Paleo," to you I say: Caveman would if he could. Whether you do is up to you.

Why would you eat Paleo when cavemen died young?

This is one objection nearly every Paleo skeptic will have, but it's easily answered. It's true that many Stone Agers died young and infant mortality rates were high at that time, but it's not because of what they were eating. Brutal conditions, club-wielding adversaries, bubbling tar pits, and no access to WebMD can really take a toll on your life span. In modern times, however, we have grocery stores, electricity, UGG boots, the Internet, running water, and emergency medical care so that when we're trampled by a mastodon we can get stitched right up. This makes it far easier to live into adulthood.

Did you hear? They found remains of ancient bread. I guess Paleo people did eat grains . . . nanny-nanny boo-boo.

A portion of this book is dedicated to dispelling the myth that grains are an important part of the human diet. (They aren't.) Unfortunately, this is the greatest sticking point for many people—people are *real* protective of their sandwiches, pizzas, and pastas, especially the "whole-grain" kind. Whenever a remnant of ancient food is discovered, it can become the subject of anti-Paleo jabs.

There are three problems with this line of thinking. First, the "ancient bread" discovered is not made with our modern, processed so-called whole grains, and it's not combined with the garbage the processed-food industry adds to its bread, pizza, and pasta. Second, ancient bread is generally composed of rhizomes—which are not grains at all but underground, root-like stems. Third, grains in general span a vast array of nutritional territory, and to truly talk about 'em, you need a lot more information than is covered in an anti-Paleo sound bite.

In the end, all the hemming and hawing over which foods are Paleo, what cavemen ate, when people started eating bread, and whether Neanderthals could play chess are merely distractions. The true point of the Paleo lifestyle is to know your food and nutrition, to understand the origins of modern nutrition myths, and to use that information to choose the types of foods that help, not harm; that aren't produced by high-profit corporations; and that have always been food.

But I read about this study . . .

The final hurdle to full Paleo enlightenment is the so-called science that is purported to prove that saturated fat, cholesterol, animal products, and other components of this lifestyle, from sunshine to salt (we'll talk about those), are dangerous.

This is perhaps the most unfortunate aspect of our modern dietary dogma. Much of the nutrition and health research over the last several decades has been done at the behest of vested interests—meaning that research is often commissioned to prove a certain predetermined idea. The government often uses inconclusive research to support its own nutrition advice, a fact brought to light by a response to the most recent government-issued "Dietary Guidelines for Americans" published by concerned scientists in the journal *Nutrition*.

Many things that should be studied are not, due to lack of funding, so even if there wasn't peer-reviewed research to support the ideas in this book (there is), a simple lack of research doesn't automatically negate a set of ideas. While it is important to be aware of current research and scientific studies to bolster our knowledge and support our own common sense, it's also important to understand exactly what we're looking at so we don't get caught with our pants—er, loincloths—down.

Though the Paleo movement is supported by good science, it's important to recognize the limitations inherent in scientific studies and published research on health and nutrition. John Ioannidis, a highly regarded physician who has held positions at Harvard, Stanford, and Tufts, authored the essay "Why Most Published Research Findings Are False" to impress upon his peers the limitations of scientific studies—most notably, how frequently studies are cited even after they are disproved. In his essay, he specifically addresses several well-known health studies that, despite having been refuted, continued to be referenced for years after they were discredited.

It's not until we understand a bit more about the "science" that we can truly know whom to trust. In short: Use scientific research wisely. I've attempted to do just that in this book.

On scientific studies

Ever said, read, or Pete-n'-repeated the phrases *studies show* or *they did a study* without actually reading the study and examining its funding, structure, design, and conclusions?

Most of us have. We assume that journalists, writers, and doctors truly grasp the full meaning of a given piece of research before they speak or write about it. Unfortunately, that's not always the case.

One of the most important things to know about the scientific research on diet that's often parroted in pop media is that whatever you're told is probably not what it seems. When it comes to the state of modern scientific inquiry, we have signed for a delivery of a big old load of bull. Here is a rundown on a few of the most glaring issues in nutritional research.

Lies, damn lies, and "relative risk"

In the chapter on fat, I talk at length about cholesterol dogma, which is one of the most deeply ingrained myths on the nutrition table. A whole division of the pharmaceutical industry revolves around combating cholesterol, and one of the most popular kinds of drugs for heart disease—statins—are said to be supported by extensive research. If you see a commercial for a statin drug, you may be told that its effectiveness nears some fantastical number—something like, say, a 33 percent "reduction in relative risk."

If someone who's terrified of heart disease was told that there's a drug that reduces the relative risk of a heart attack by 33 percent, he'd probably take it. But would he first ask what "relative risk" means?

If he did, he might change his mind.

Shane Ellison, a former pharmaceutical drug chemist, reveals what the concept truly means in his book *Hidden Truth about Cholesterol-Lowering Drugs*. Relative risk, in this case, is simply the difference—expressed as a percentage—between the outcomes observed in two different groups. Let's say a group that takes statins is being compared to one that takes a placebo pill. Out of one hundred people in the statin group, two—2 percent—have a heart attack. Out of one hundred people in the placebo group, three—3 percent—have a heart attack. Comparing these two groups, you'd think that the difference in the incidence of heart attacks between the two groups would be just 1 percent, which could as easily be due to coincidence as it could be to effective medication.

Is 1 percent enough of a difference to make you take a medication with a wide range of side effects, including deep muscle pain and memory loss?

Probably not. So, instead of advertising that measly 1 percent, drug companies do something tricky: They massage the numbers. Since the difference between a 3 percent risk and a 2 percent risk is 1 percent, and 1 percent is one-third of 3 percent, they state that their product offers a 33 percent reduction in *relative* risk. Suddenly, 1 percent becomes 33 percent, and the cost-benefit ratio of taking a statin starts to look pretty darn good.

And then they drown your puppy and cancel your Netflix subscription.

These are the self-serving tricks drug companies play to make their stuff sound good. Yes, this practice is legal— or, at least, it's not *illegal*—and yes, it's done with alarming frequency.

Relative risk isn't the only research tool that should make us go hmm. One of the most common methods for studying diet and health is the *dietary recall*.

Do you recall what you had for breakfast last year? Yeah, me neither.

Many of the most frequently cited nutrition studies are dietary recall studies. These studies may be done on small groups, or they may be used in "cohort studies" of extremely large populations. Surveys are given to individuals who are expected to remember what they ate on a daily basis so that researchers can investigate possible connections between diet and the incidence of certain diseases. Sometimes participants fill out these surveys on a daily basis for more accurate reporting (who remembers what they ate last week?), but sometimes the surveys require an accurate memory of months and years of past habits. Regardless of how frequently the surveys are filled out—whether immediately after a meal or weeks, even months, later—dietary recall studies are infamously unreliable for two reasons: recall bias and response bias. *Recall bias* refers to the fact that many people don't have an accurate memory of what they've eaten, and *response bias* refers to our propensity to lie, skew the truth, or delude ourselves about what, and how much, we eat.

Do you remember what you had for breakfast last Tuesday? And if you did, would you even want to admit to what you ate?

Even the Food and Agriculture Organization of the United Nations admits that survey studies of worldwide nutrition data "all suffer from a degree of underreporting. This can be intentional or involuntary, most likely due to individuals forgetting food items or not describing foods thought to be undesirable."

Correlation is not causation

Another challenge of modern nutrition research is the "correlation versus causation" pitfall. These are totally different concepts, but they're often conflated. *Correlation* means that two variables have been observed in the same set of data; however, it does not mean that one variable directly causes the other. *Causation* does mean that one variable causes another. It's rare that causation is proved at all; many studies merely report correlative data.

For example, if I observe that countries where people eat lots of broccoli also have high rates of foot fungus, would it be reasonable to assume that broccoli *causes* foot fungus? Or could something else be at work?

Just because broccoli intake and foot fungus are observed in the same set of data does not mean that eating broccoli causes someone to develop foot fungus. Yet this set of data could be reported in a manner that sounds an awful lot like causation to a layperson: "Broccoli consumption *is correlated with* foot fungus." "Broccoli consumption *is associated with* foot fungus." "Broccoli consumption *increases the risk of* foot fungus."

This certainly sounds ridiculous, but it's the same logic that is often applied to studies on nutrition variables. We'll encounter this problem several times in this book, including in the discussions of fat and salt. A population study may indicate that chronically high blood pressure is observed with high frequency in populations that eat high amounts of salt, but that doesn't mean—as much as we might like to believe it—that eating some salt *causes chronically* high blood pressure. On the contrary, these populations may eat most of their salt in the form of processed food filled with not just salt but also damaged fats, refined sugar, and artificial preservatives. There are confounding factors, then, that make this association less valid, as the damaged fats, refined sugar, and artificial preservatives could play a part just as easily as salt. In the example about broccoli consumption, a high incidence of foot fungus could be a result of confounding factors like a desire to eat more healthfully in an attempt to heal foot fungus naturally; the fact that broccoli is eaten most in developed countries, where sweaty shoes and gym locker rooms incubate fungi, enabling fungi to thrive; or even—and most likely—pure coincidence.

Beyond that, many studies attempt to isolate certain nutrients to blame them for disease or laud them for their supposedly positive effect on health. As you'll see repeatedly throughout this book, assessing the effects of nutrients *in isolation* completely disregards the way nutrients work together in nature. Look for the word *synergy*. (Never mock synergy.)

While there are far more scientific pitfalls that those I've listed here, the overall caution is this: Unless we're aware of how a study is funded, designed, conducted, summarized, and finally reported, phrased, and spun, we can't always know what its conclusions really mean. And it's even harder to get at the truth when we read about a study secondhand, thirdhand, or fifthhand in a news article, e-mail blast, or online report.

This is why I am interested in scientific studies but am rarely convinced by their conclusions alone, whether they affirm my own prejudices or not (though I have to say, many of them *do* support my claims). Today's fallible studies on diet and health have distracted us from looking at what else matters when it comes to food: how food works in the body (biology), what we evolved to eat (evolutionary biology), the long-standing record of what humans ate for millennia (anthropology), and, of course, the forgotten science of common sense, which takes into account the history of today's nutrition dogma and the silly, often shady dealings behind it. While it's incredibly hard to meld all these disciplines into a well-composed "big picture," there are several professionals who dedicate their lives to synthesizing all the research, science, history, and common sense—and they are cited in this book.

So here's where we stand, and here's where we're going

My interests extend far beyond simply confirming that Paleo principles work. I've also learned that it's not just about what you do and don't eat; it's about knowing why. It's about choosing the foods with the best nutrition and expanding the scope of "what would a caveman do" to "which real foods have the most nutrients and the longest history in the human diet." It's not about dogma; it's about knowledge. It's about choosing food that makes sense to your body, mind, and soul. It's about the intersection between good science, history, and common sense.

The way we think about eating and health is completely and utterly broken. We've been lied to more than once, and these lies have been popularized, propagandized, and painstakingly ingrained in our culture.

We've lost sight of what we really need to be healthy and happy: real, nutrient-dense food. The kind of food that balances the body and the mind. The kind of food that has been nourishing humans for thousands of years. We don't need more dogma or another diet plan. We need *nutrition*.

We also need a nice whack of truth that can be rubbed in Uncle Ed's face at Thanksgiving dinner when he tells us that choosing butter rather than margarine will give us heart attacks. (It won't.)

The modern nutrition world is a minefield of meticulously crafted lies. And when we dig deeper, we find—hiding in plain sight—the evidence of decades of industry influence, twisted science, and health hype that has sent us down a path of sheer frustration and confusion. And it's not going to end until we uncover the truth.

Of course, simply saying "we've been lied to" as justification for a sweeping shift in what we eat is like trying to defuse a bomb with a pair of travel tweezers. It's a necessary piece of the puzzle and an intriguing sound bite, but it's not enough. What we really need is information. All the information we can squeeze into one place, so that we can learn how the heck we got here and why we need a change, and, from there, armed with knowledge and confidence in a new way of life, decide how we should move forward.

Let's get to it.

Chapter 1

....

fat

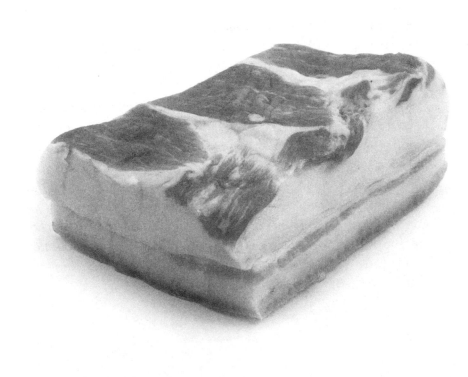

Fat.

There are few words as unsettling.

Say it out loud. Does the word fall from your lips melodiously, wrapped in silken threads of happiness? Does it roll across your tongue like raindrops on a lily pad?

Of course not. It punches its way across your psyche and, if you believe the hype, leaves clogged arteries in its wake.

Why? Because we've spent decades believing that dietary fat is the enemy. Where we once embraced foods rich in natural fat, we now obsess over what the fat in our food is going to do to our hearts and our cholesterol levels. We decided—probably because we heard it from someone who heard it from someone else, whether a doctor, a pharmaceutical rep, or an actor in a Cheerios commercial—that dietary fat is just as bad as body fat, and we spend our lives avoiding the foods rich in the types of dietary fat that nourished human beings for thousands of years before bad science demonized them.

Specifically, we avoid foods rich in natural saturated fat and cholesterol. We avoid a nice, rare steak. We throw away egg yolks. We test our blood cholesterol levels to make sure that our strategy is working.

But it's not working. Despite all the fat-lowering and cholesterol-obsessing, people are still sick with the same diseases that those changes were supposed to prevent. And when rigorous studies and trials like the Nurses Health Study and the Women's Health Initiative Dietary Modification Trial failed to show that a low-fat diet has any benefits for long-term health, the powers that be began giving a few types of fats a hall pass: specifically fats from plants, like highly profitable plant-based oils. (Oils are simply fats in liquid form.)

The most common dietary plant-based oils, like soybean oil, corn oil, and canola oil, are certainly politically correct: They're free of the baggage surrounding saturated fat and animal products. They're the fats from which margarine is usually made. They're highly profitable. They're also highly processed and totally unfit for human consumption.

For the sake of differentiating these types of plant oils from the healthy, whole, fat-containing plants I do consider healthful (avocados, coconuts, nuts, and olives), let's call them *crop oils*—partially because they're derived from big-profit agricultural crops, and partially because the word *crop* looks a lot like the word *crap,* and I like that.

These crop oils are sometimes called *seed oils,* but they are most often referred to as, and labeled, *vegetable oils.* Although the association with vegetables certainly makes these oils sound healthy, the truth is quite the opposite: They're not at all healthy, and they're not made from vegetables. Corn is a grain, not a vegetable. Soybeans are legumes, not vegetables. Canola oil is derived from a seed, not a vegetable. Cottonseed oil is derived from cotton, not a vegetable.

By contrast, the fat in natural, unprocessed food, especially saturated fat, is one of the most amazing things on this planet. The same goes for cholesterol.

Saturated fat is abundant in animal products. Cholesterol is found only in animal products. And this is not what's scary about animal products. It's what *special* about them.

Yet we've been told not to trust saturated fat and cholesterol. We've been told they'll hurt—even kill—us. Many vegans and vegetarians have eliminated animal products from their diets because of this unfounded fear.

And that's been a very convenient state of affairs for the status quo. We've built our entire zeitgeist around it. The pharmaceutical, weight-loss, food, and fitness industries—and all the television shows, magazines, books, and websites associated with them—depend on it.

The hodgepodge of jackassery and lies that stitch together health fears, nutrition dogma, and profitable products disguised as health foods is damn difficult to tease apart. But if we don't try, well, who's the *real* jackass?

Let's talk about fat, baby

Everything we've been told about the dangers of fat and cholesterol is wrong. Wrong like airplane food. Wrong like a pair of acid-washed manpris.

Let's usher in a new era. Let's move on. But first, let's dunk decades of conventional wisdom and heart disease hoodwinkery in a great big vat of pork fat.

In other words: Damn the man. Save the bacon drippings.

If you've been staying away from natural fat and choking down highly processed substitutes for the real thing, I've got some amazing news: Natural, unrefined fat is perfectly healthy. Especially fat from properly raised animals. So make yourself a latte, pour in the cream, and enjoy your three-egg omelet with all the yolks. Your body, your skin, and your brain will thank you.

Natural, healthy fat is your friend—and a damn good one at that. It's the kind of friend that's straightforward, does what's best for you, and comes with benefits that'll make you want to take your relationship to the next level.

Relationship status: It's not complicated!

We *need* healthy fat. We need cholesterol, too. I'd go so far as to say that we don't need to eat more plants (although plants of the fruit-and-vegetable variety are certainly not going to hurt anybody); we need to eat more natural *fats.*

Healthy fats come in many varieties, and when we truly understand their structures and the roles they play in keeping our bodies and minds healthy, there's not much else to say but "Can you cook that in lard, please?"

Oh, and one more thing, in case the point wasn't clear: Fat does not make you fat. The first red flag about that old myth? That the rise of obesity in America began right as fat and cholesterol were all-out demonized and has continued through decades of low-fat diets and fat-free factory foods.

Fact is, we *need* fat. This point is nonnegotiable. A review coauthored by Walter Willett, chair of the department of nutrition at the Harvard School of Public Health, included the explosive statement that "It is now increasingly recognized that the low-fat campaign has been based on little scientific evidence and may have caused unintended health consequences."

I'll translate: When it comes to a low-fat diet, we totally missed the nutritional boat. Scratch that—we screwed the pooch every which way from Sunday.

That the low-fat dogma had unintended consequences is not at all surprising considering that our bodies need fat to utilize fat-soluble vitamins, which are *everything* to our health. Fat also stabilizes the appetite by affecting satiety hormones, which make us feel full. Fat does not trigger insulin release the way sugar does. Fat provides long-burning, consistent energy that carbohydrates just can't match. Fat makes our cells strong. We need different types of fats, because different types of fats provide different nutrients and different cell-building materials.

So it's important to understand this stuff—first, so we can eat the right fats; and second, so we can be smarter than everybody else. (That's not a joke.)

Let's start by defining our terms. What do we mean when we talk about fat, anyway? What are the different kinds of fat, and why do they matter?

To really understand what fat is all about, we need some formal training in fatty acids

When we talk about fat types—*saturated, monounsaturated,* and *polyunsaturated*—we're actually talking about fatty acids. Fatty acids are chains of carbon and hydrogen atoms attached to a carboxyl group, which is like a hinge that keeps the individual chains together. Every fat, whether plant or animal, is made up of those same raw materials.

In a saturated fat, every link in the fatty acid chain is secured—it's *saturated.* (Lightbulb!) This means it's strong, resistant to oxidative damage, and stable. Monounsaturated fats have just one unsecured link (*mono* means *one*). Polyunsaturated fats have two or more unsecured links in their chains.

In truth, almost all the natural fats we eat are a blend of these three kinds of fats. Lard, for example, contains some saturated fats, some monounsaturated fats, and some polyunsaturated fats. So does butter. So does olive oil, which is famous for just one of the three fats it contains: monounsaturated fat, which, as I mentioned, is also found in lard.

Head spinning? Just remember, whatever a fat is *mostly* made of—whether saturated, monounsaturated, or polyunsaturated—is generally what we call it. It's tyranny of the majority. Olive oil is *mostly* monounsaturated, so that's what we call it, even though it also contains saturated fat. Lard is called *saturated* even though it has just slightly less saturated fat than monounsaturated.

We've been led to believe that plant fats are vastly different from animal fats. This is partly true, but not for the reasons we think.

Depending on how the links in these chains are put together, combining a whole mess of hinged-up chains may yield what we label a *fat,* which is generally solid at room temperature (like butter), or an *oil,* which is generally liquid at room temperature.

Whatever the term, we're talking about the same raw materials—fatty acids—so whether I use the word *fat* or the word *oil*, I'm talking about the same building blocks.

So here's the God's honest truth: Animal fats don't have extra-dangerous, heart-attacking gremlins hidden between their hydrogen atoms. These are the same ol' hydrogen and carbon atoms found in plants, people, and everything else on this planet.

The fat- and cholesterol-rich foods that healthy humans ate for hundreds, even thousands, of years deserve a little freakin' credit. And we owe it to ourselves not only to understand what makes those foods so great but also to figure out how we managed to forget centuries of history in favor of decades of unproven theories. What the heck happened?

History and the heart

Think about how rumors get started. One person says something to another, who repeats it to another, and as the message hums along, it takes on a life of its own. People use it for their own gain. It's unstoppable—and now, with the constant chirp of social media, rumors have gone from controlled blazes to raging wildfires.

Picture this: Sally tells Jimmy that fat and cholesterol are bad and cause heart disease. Jimmy starts a multijillion-dollar company that sells fat-free whoozits, low-fat whatzits, and cholesterol-free thingamabobs. Sally tells Jimmy she might have been wrong. Jimmy unfriends her on Facebook.

That's an oversimplification. But in the history of the demonization of fats and cholesterol, it's not too far from the truth.

Fear of cholesterol and fat springs in large part from our fear of heart disease. The two concepts have grown together like the hair in a hippie's dreadlocks: If we want to avoid heart disease, we'd damn well better eliminate those gall-darned lipids. (Ha! Biliary joke!)

The heart disease epidemic is a relatively new problem in human history. The first recorded heart attack was in 1912. By 1930, the number of deaths from heart attacks had reached over 3,000, and come 1960, there were over 500,000 recorded deaths from heart attacks. People were terrified. They needed an explanation, and they needed something to blame.

That cultural panic led to the development of two theories that became imprinted on the collective consciousness: the lipid hypothesis and the diet-heart hypothesis.

The lipid hypothesis contends that high cholesterol in the blood causes, or at the very least guarantees, heart disease. This idea is the foundation of the pharmaceutical industry's production of their most profitable drugs, statins, and underlies our cultural obsession with lipid panels and cholesterol testing. Oh, and incidentally—it's a load of hooey.

The diet-heart hypothesis contends that the saturated fat and cholesterol that we eat increase blood cholesterol levels, and because high blood cholesterol supposedly increases the risk of heart disease (hello, lipid hypothesis hooey), dietary saturated fat and cholesterol must therefore cause heart attacks. This is also a load of hooey.

That's how fat—especially the saturated animal fat that had been part of the human diet for millennia—was wrongly accused, falsely convicted, and sent to the guillotine. Picture the townspeople storming the castle in Disney's *Beauty and the Beast*. That's pretty much what happened to fat, especially animal fat. It was hunted down and demonized, and there was no princess to kiss it all better (and no talking candlestick to illuminate the truth, for that matter).

Unfortunately, the sad story behind the long-term survival of these hypotheses is not just one of good intentions gone awry. It's also one of data mismanagement, selective memory, corporate greed, and a bit of see-what-you-want-to-see.

The problems with the hypotheses

Let's start here: In 1954, a researcher fed some cholesterol to rabbits. The rabbits developed arterial damage. This researcher did not, however, prove that this is also what happens in humans. Because, like, it *doesn't*. In fact, you might even say that rabbits and humans are entirely different animals.

Rabbits—tiny herbivores not designed by nature to consume cholesterol-rich foods like meat, eggs, and butter—have completely different metabolic machinery than humans. A rabbit with a cholesterol problem simply doesn't translate to a human with a heart issue.

The same researcher, in a separate endeavor, showed that polyunsaturated fats (like those from soybean or corn oil) could, in the right context, lower blood cholesterol in humans.

But, as I'll discuss in more detail later, someone with low blood cholesterol does not, statistically, have a lower risk of heart disease. So even if eating polyunsaturated fat appears to lower blood cholesterol, that doesn't mean it will also prevent a heart attack. That's a leap of logic we're far too used to making—and one that has more holes than a pair of Crocs.

So are the results of these studies really enough to convince you that eating cholesterol gives people heart disease and eating corn oil prevents heart attacks? I certainly hope not, although they convinced enough folks to ruin lard for the rest of us.

Interestingly, lipid biochemist Mary Enig believes that polyunsaturated fats might appear to lower cholesterol because they are incorporated into cell membranes, weakening them to the point that cholesterol—which the body uses for cell repair—is recruited out of the blood to stabilize them.

According to Chris Masterjohn, an expert in nutrition science, randomized, controlled trials have shown that polyunsaturated fats cannot reduce heart disease. In fact, *no* study on replacing animal fats with plant-based polyunsaturated fat has shown a reduction in mortality. Masterjohn has stated that these studies "showed an increased risk of cancer after five years and a possible increase in heart disease risk."

Knowing all this, the natural conclusion is, of course, to build an entire empire of factory-made fats like "heart-healthy" polyunsaturated "vegetable" oils made from highly processed corn, soybeans, and canola.

That's sarcasm. Why? Because corn is a grain, not a vegetable. Soybeans are legumes, not vegetables. Canola is derived from a seed, not a vegetable, and though it is not as high in polyunsaturated fat as corn or soybean oil, it is just as highly processed.

Sigh.

Correlation is not causation, remember?

Next in line for the data dunce cap is Ancel Keys, who was named to the board of the American Heart Association (an organization that has relied heavily on donations from the crop oil industry) in the late 1950s. Keys's nutritional qualifications were slim and specific: He had created the army's K-ration, kissing cousin to today's MRE.

This is not an encouraging testament to his experience with real, unprocessed foods.

Keys published his own observational data—meaning, he wrote up his personal observations and dressed them up as science—on a few trends he observed in several cultures regarding their food supply and rates of heart disease. He insisted that populations with more access to dietary fat tend to have more deaths from heart disease. Although this wasn't what his data actually showed, it was how he chose to present it.

If you recall our discussion of correlation and causation from the introduction, you'll understand why these kinds of observations often carry about as much weight as a wet paper bag. There are too many factors at work in life to assume that two variables observed in the same place at the same time are automatically related.

For example, as noted earlier, if I observe that countries where people eat lots of broccoli also have high rates of foot fungus, would it be reasonable to assume that broccoli causes foot fungus? Or could something else be at work? By the same token, just because a country has a lot of dietary fat in its food supply does not mean that the fat is responsible for that country's health concerns. Before it became ingrained in our minds that fat is something to be feared, the whole notion would have seemed as ridiculous as cruciferous vegetable–induced athlete's foot.

Keys engaged in some data deception by failing to acknowledge the mountain of evidence that didn't support his own theories. Because he was a hammer and fat was the nail, Keys failed to notice—or perhaps purposely ignored—data that would have hurt his hypothesis or that suggested entirely different causes of heart disease.

Remember: Correlation is not causation. People in wealthier countries—those with more access to luxuries like televisions, cars, and rich, nutrient-dense, fat-filled foods—also have access to other excesses, especially foods high in sugar and poor in nutrients, which dentist and nutrition researcher Weston A. Price called the "foods of commerce."

And let's be honest. Almost any time we blame foods high in fat for health problems, we're talking about foods that are also high in carbs and refined sugar: Doughnuts. Cakes. Candy. Breaded, deep-fried fast foods.

Price, who observed the dietary customs of native cultures around the world, identified cultures with diets rich in fat and cholesterol as the healthiest of all. In fact, he observed such diets to be universally health-promoting. But he also saw disease and degeneration as cultures embraced a diet high in white flour and sugar and reduced their consumption of traditional foods, such as animal products and seafood.

Could Price's observations be considered just another Keys-like problem of correlation versus causation? Perhaps. But here's the difference: Biology. Science. Nutrition. The foods Price's thriving cultures enjoyed were part of these healthy people's diets for generations upon healthy, fertile generations, and they contained the nutrients that play important roles in cellular health, bodily function, mental health, and even satiety signaling. (More on this as the chapter rolls on.) Compare that to the average American diet over the last fifty years of the low-fat movement. Eating low-fat, highly processed food has just made us fatter and sicker.

Although other scientists publicly lambasted Keys for the glaring lack of evidence in support of his theory, the powers that were—prominent business executives and influential scientists with ties to the crop oil industry, including those making up the board of the American Heart Association at that time—were overwhelmingly committed to promoting the poorly constructed theory that humans are better off with less fat and cholesterol in our diet.

This chain of events led many to call Keys the "Father of the Low-Fat Diet." Ouch, says the butter-lover.

America turns away from natural fats

In *The Oiling of America*, a scathing exposé of the false demonization of natural fats and the false deification of low-cholesterol diets rich in crop oils, Enig traces the intertwining of certain influential scientists with the crop oil industry. In 1956, a diet low in saturated fat and cholesterol and high in these newfangled crop oils was advocated publicly by Irving Page and Jeremiah Stamler in a televised fund-raiser for the American Heart Association. These same men, along with Keys, would go on to design the AHA nutritional guidelines of 1961.

The principles advocated by Page and Stamler came to compose the "prudent diet," which was based on the AHA dogma promoting a diet low in cholesterol and high in poly-unsaturated fats from crop oils. So confident was the crop oil industry in this diet that corporations like Wesson and Mazola began touting the yet-unproven health benefits of their products to the public that same year. Premature? Probably. Profitable? Absolutely.

The anti-saturated-fat, anti-cholesterol message was becoming ingrained in the American mind. And we were steadily forgetting the types of foods we'd eaten in good health for centuries.

Fast-forward to 1984, when results from a nonstatin cholesterol-lowering drug trial showed, according to Masterjohn, that removing damaged lipids from the body lowers the risk of heart disease. (We'll talk about damaged lipids later.) *Time* magazine took this to mean that reducing the cholesterol we eat by avoiding cholesterol-rich foods would also lower the risk of heart disease. Of course, the trial had proved nothing of the sort. Cholesterol in food, as we'll discuss, has very little bearing on blood cholesterol. The two are entirely different things.

Yet *Time* magazine found this distinction irrelevant, and its March 26, 1984, cover showed bacon and eggs shaped into the creative bummer of the century: a fatty breakfast frowny face composed of two over-easy eyes and a sad pork-belly pout. Cholesterol in food, it said, was "deadly." The country descended into fat-phobic, cholesterol-counting hysteria.

It was officially a runaway train, one that George V. Mann, former director of the longest-running heart-health study, later called "the greatest biomedical error of the twentieth century."

By this time, representatives from the crop oil industry—the folks whose margarine and corn, soybean, and canola oils were becoming staples in every kitchen—had obtained positions in the Food and Drug Administration, the American Medical Association, the American Heart Association, the National Cholesterol Education Program, and the Senate Select Committee on Nutrition and Human Needs.

This could only mean one thing: Crop oils and margarine were here to stay.

And so were a few public health nuisances, such as obesity and heart disease. Obesity in adults more than doubled between 1980 and 2008, and "extreme obesity" more than quadrupled. Heart disease and stroke remain the leading causes of death in the United States today, and obesity-related disease has replaced starvation as the world's greatest risk to health.

We had our bogeyman in fat and cholesterol, yet America's health just got worse. So who was the *real* bad guy? And why the scapegoating of natural, traditional foods like eggs, cream, and red meat?

What really causes heart disease?

Unfortunately for those who want easy answers and something to blame, heart disease—and most other modern health epidemics, for that matter—probably results from a combination of factors, from the moment it takes root to the moment it kills. There is no one villain, but the problem certainly is not the traditional foods that humans have eaten for centuries.

Researchers have pointed to sugar, stress, nutrient deficiency, nutrient imbalance, rancid or damaged fats (like those from processed crop oils), smoking, and the chronic inflammation that results from all of the above as major contributing factors in heart disease. The oxidation of lipoproteins—that is, damage to the molecules that carry cholesterol, not to cholesterol itself—and the length of time those molecules linger in the body may also contribute to the development of heart disease. These factors are influenced by things like stress and nutrient deficiency.

Insulin resistance—a precursor to diabetes, another modern-day health epidemic—is also a telltale sign of heart disease risk. Lipidology experts Thomas Dayspring and James A. Underberg cite dietary carbohydrates, especially fructose and high-fructose corn syrup, as common instigators of insulin resistance. Most of us already know that high-fructose corn syrup is dangerous, but carbohydrates in general? Aren't carbs supposed to be healthy?

Think about this: The anti–saturated fat, anti-cholesterol, pro–crop oil movement spawned innumerable industries and companies that produce processed foods low in cholesterol and saturated fat but rich in carbohydrates that were never known to humanity in the thousands of years prior. Isn't it possible that the processed foods that filled the butter-free void are at least indirectly responsible for our contemporary heart-related health crisis?

And if that's the case, then what new foods were we eating before these processed foods existed, when heart disease first began its steady climb? (Remember, we ate saturated-fat-filled animal foods for millennia before heart disease became a public health problem, so let's look elsewhere for an answer.)

The problem may have been something that entered our food supply long before modern processed junk compounded the problem: trans fats.

Trans fats: The nightmare continues

The consumption of partially hydrogenated oils, which began in the early 1900s and increased during World War II, may have played a major role in the development of the heart disease epidemic—long before we began blaming saturated fat and cholesterol.

Partial hydrogenation involves hardening an oil, or any fat that softens at room temperature, into a never-melts, never-moves, odorless, tasteless solid (think Crisco) to increase its shelf life and—yes, this is a real industry word—plasticity. (Yep, these used to be called *plastic fats*.) Partially hydrogenating the liquid fats from soybean oil, corn oil, and canola oil only adds to their long process of refinement. The process of partial hydrogenation involves forcing hydrogen into an oil's structure using a chemical catalyst. The miracle of science, right?

That little miracle is also where trans fats come from.

Trans fats are created as a result of the partial hydrogenation process. Or, as I like to describe it, the process of beating an already unhealthy oil into partially hydrogenated submission.

Why make a solid fat out of an oil? Because many cheap commodity oils, especially crop oils, are uniquely fragile and vulnerable to damage. Once solidified, they are less likely to spoil. So, as an alternative to spoilage, we create frankenfats with a different chemical structure than any natural fat humans have ever eaten. Brilliant.

Here's the science behind what makes trans fats dangerous, from Enig:

> *When one hydrogen atom is moved to the other side of the fatty acid molecule during hydrogenation, the ability of living cells to make reactions at the site is compromised or altogether lost . . . . [Trans fats'] altered chemical structure creates havoc with thousands of necessary chemical reactions—everything from energy provision to prostaglandin production.*

If you've seen as many Will Smith movies as I have, you'll recall the scene in *Men in Black* where Edgar, an undeniable jerk, is killed and his body inhabited by a giant alien cockroach hell-bent on destroying the world.

Think of pre-cockroach Edgar as a crop oil: a jerk whose existence makes the world worse, but not something as horrifying as, say, the *Saw* movie franchise. Now, think of alien cockroach Edgar as a trans fat–filled, partially hydrogenated crop oil: an evil, barely recognizable, fundamentally altered, dangerous version of his old self who will seek you out and destroy you.

Trans fats are cockroaches in Edgar suits. They're so poisonous, in fact—they're associated with cancer, heart disease, inflammation, and infertility—that the Food and Drug Administration finally considered banning them beginning in 2013.

It's important to note, though, that artificial trans fats generated through partial hydrogenation are the ones causing problems. These human-made trans fats have a different chemical structure than a naturally occurring trans fat called *conjugated linoleic acid* (CLA), which is created in the digestive system of grazing animals. CLA is found in the fat of these animals and is widely known to fight cancer and support metabolism. We can think of human-made trans fats from partially hydrogenated oils as the evil doppelgängers of CLA.

Trans fats, as you can see, hide behind terms like *partially hydrogenated,* and words like liquid shortening and *fractionated* may indicate equally harsh processing. The creation of a solid fat from a liquid oil is right up there with Dr. Frankenstein's monster as a science experiment that never should have happened. Think about it. Churning cream for a short time makes butter. Churning soybean oil for a year wouldn't make margarine, yet the Moreau-like insanity of the processed-food industry manages to make it happen.

Unfortunately, the FDA only began requiring the labeling of trans fat–containing foods in 2006, and there were loopholes—less than 0.5 gram of trans fat per serving in a given food meant that a food manufacturer could still label it "trans fat free." (Quick note: Isn't there something *off* about the term *food manufacturer*?) Crisco, for example, has proudly declared itself to have "0 g trans fats," yet as of 2013 was still using partially hydrogenated oils. That phrase—*partially hy-drogenated oils*—is the truth-teller, because where there are partially hydrogenated oils, there are always trans fats.

See why they're so insidious? They avoid detection even today, when their dangers are recognized.

For many years, margarine had high levels of trans fats since it was made with partially hydrogenated oils. Shortening has long been made with partially hydrogenated oils—even the butter-flavored versions, which, of course, contain no but-ter. Here's why that matters: The rate of heart disease in the United States increased as consumption of margarine and shortening increased from the early 1900s on. Coincidence?

This could mean it wasn't natural saturated fat or choles-terol that pushed our health to the danger zone in the first place but, instead, artificially solidified, partially hydroge-nated, trans fat–rich foods derived from crop oils, with all the earmarks of mad-scientist spawn.

Out of the frying pan, into the partially hydrogenated fire.

Interestingly, even Keys agreed that trans fats were a like-ly culprit in heart disease. But even though Keys was an in-dustry insider, his stance didn't prompt a shift back to tradi-tional fats derived from butter, cream, or red meat. It simply pushed the crop oil industry further down its own cornhole. Margarine, corn oil, and shortening companies began fund-ing research intended to prove that saturated fat from ani-mal sources was dangerous, leading to propaganda meant to convince us that the natural saturated fats found in ani-mals were somehow worse than what they were making in factories.

All together now: Seriously?!

The American Heart Association, furthering its reputa-tion as an instrument of the crop oil industry, removed all references to the potential negative effects of trans fats from the 1968 recommendations of its Subcommittee on Dietary Fats at the urging of the Shortening Institute, now known as the Institute of Shortening and Edible Oils, a group whose website boasts that its members produce "approximately 90–95% of the edible fats and oils produced domestically (28 billion pounds)," including shortening, margarine, and cooking oils. Two words underlie that statement: *power* and *influence*.

This trans fat malfeasance was revealed by a member of the very committee that worked on those recommendations: Fred A. Kummerow, a professor of food chemistry at the University of Illinois, who today is a passionate saturated-fat activist. In a 1977 letter to Senator George McGovern, then-chairman of the Select Committee on Nutrition and Human Needs, Kummerow condemned the decade-long failure of the FDA and the National Institutes of Health (NIH) to do anything about the public health hazard of trans fats.

The propaganda supporting trans fats had worked, crop oils were a permanent fixture in the American diet, and myths and dogma about saturated fat and heart disease rolled on.

Irony: When "healthy" foods make you sick

One thing's for sure: Animal fat and the cholesterol-rich, saturated fat–filled natural foods that people enjoyed in good health for thousands of years are not the dirty birds in this wild goose chase.

In fact, Americans were eating fewer animal fats and more crop oils, most notably partially hydrogenated crop oils, as rates of heart disease increased between 1900 and the 1950s. According to psychotherapist Judith Shaw in her book *Trans Fats: The Hidden Killer in Our Food*, at the same time saturated fat was implicated in the heart disease epidemic, "USDA figures showed that butter consumption in the

United States had actually dropped to one-quarter of what it had been at the turn of the century while consumption of hydrogenated vegetable oil margarine had risen 200 percent."

Common sense suggests that animal fats couldn't possibly be the problem. Luckily for margarine, however, common sense is about as rare as clothing on a French beach. Perhaps that's why I used to stock my own fridge with fake butter and my cabinet with canola oil and Crisco, and why I was so sure that a single bite of rib eye would end up fused to my arteries.

The dietary advice and drug prescriptions we've been given since fat and cholesterol fell (or, more accurately, were shoved, battered, and beaten) out of fashion have not decreased the incidence of heart disease. Or cancer. Or stroke. Or obesity. This is one reason that today's medical system is so overwhelmed and the health care sector is one of the few growing industries in these tough economic times.

The Centers for Disease Control (CDC) counts heart disease among "the most widespread and costly health problems facing our nation today." While you may hear the false-victory claim that deaths from heart disease have decreased, that's not because we've stopped heart disease from happening. It happens more than ever. Deaths from heart disease have decreased because we now have the technology to keep sick folks alive—even though the dietary recommendations and medical care provided to them haven't done what they should do: keep them healthy in the first place.

But with just a little perspective on nutrition and history we can see, as clear as Crystal Pepsi, that natural saturated fat and cholesterol deserve a lot more love than fifty years of blind faith in a corrupt establishment have allowed. The question of what fat means for our health deserves some serious clarification. And a few of our fatty-acid friends deserve a welcome-back parade.

Let's continue our fact-finding extravaganza with the truth about that scary substance that everybody loves to dread: cholesterol.

Cholesterol: Don't hate!

Do you know people with high cholesterol?

You may want to congratulate them. You'll definitely want to keep them from freaking out. And, so they don't think you're completely nuts, you may want to give them this book.

A cascade of evidence—not conspiracy theories but published and even peer-reviewed evidence—reveals the crazed, dated, *soooo* 1956 fear of both dietary and blood cholesterol for what it really is: total twaddle. That's a nice way of saying *bullshit*.

In fact, studies show that people with high cholesterol actually tend to be healthier and live longer than those with low cholesterol.

What we think we know about cholesterol and heart disease is little more than an overtrusted, underproven, overly simplistic view of what's actually going on in our bodies. Cholesterol simply isn't the danger that many folks—doctors included—think it is.

Let's spank the conventional cholesterol wisdom, starting with several important points. First, I encourage ample use of mental "finger quotes" with the classifications of "low" and "high" cholesterol. These terms are based on outdated, irrational standards, and the threshold for high cholesterol has dropped progressively lower over the years—a strategy that hasn't affected our success in fighting heart disease but definitely helps sell statins.

Second, cholesterol in food does not equate to cholesterol in the blood. If, after reading this book, you dare to throw away an egg yolk because you're concerned about cholesterol, know this: You made me cry. And it was an ugly cry.

Dietary and blood cholesterol share a few more characteristics, one of which is total, underappreciated badassery. Think of Old Man Marley from the classic flick *Home Alone*.

Everyone is deathly afraid of the guy, but, in the end, he's just a misunderstood old dude. And despite all the prejudice against him, he still manages to save the day by walloping the Wet Bandits with a snow shovel.

Cholesterol is a lifesaving, health-promoting substance, and it performs incredibly important functions in the body. Every one of our cells needs it at every stage of our lives, whether we're talking in the diet or in the blood. So, while dietary cholesterol is a totally separate entity from that lab-tested number the doctor wants you to reduce, both concepts are due for a major PR makeover.

Cholesterol in your food

Does the cholesterol in your food affect the amount of cholesterol in your blood? Not really. And even if it did, the fact remains that cholesterol is so necessary that the body is able to produce the stuff on its own.

"When we eat more cholesterol, the body produces less," says nutritionist and physician Natasha Campbell-McBride. "When we eat less cholesterol, the body produces more." Why eat cholesterol-rich foods, then, if the body will produce it anyway? Because it eases the body's burden and is associated with improved cognitive function, and because, in many individuals, cholesterol synthesis is inadequate for all the body's needs.

Mother Nature seems to be aware of this, so she's stacked many of the foods humans have eaten throughout history with not just cholesterol but also flavor and nourishment. Naturally cholesterol-rich foods like egg yolks, butter, meat, and seafood are packaged with other powerful nutrients, like vitamins A, D, E, and K; choline; and other hormone-building, health-supporting substances, like healthy fats and minerals, that we need from infancy through old age.

Mother Nature's no dingbat. She didn't package the good stuff with bad stuff so she could watch us struggle for thousands of years until the invention of Egg Beaters. In fact, we're designed so that we get plenty of cholesterol from day one, even before we're old enough for steak and hollandaise sauce. Human breast milk is high in cholesterol because babies need plenty of it to develop healthy brains and sharp eyesight. In fact, breast milk even contains a special enzyme ensuring that babies absorb as much cholesterol as possible.

Cholesterol in your blood

According to Ellison, a former pharmaceutical drug chemist who now works to expose the dangers of indiscriminate statin use, "High cholesterol in those over 75 years of age is protective rather than harmful. . . . Low cholesterol is a risk factor for heart arrhythmia, the leading cause of death if heart attack occurs."

Yet the research and medical communities don't see any red flags or warning signs in the standard cholesterol dogma—probably because it's all they know, and because it's a large chunk of what they get paid for. When researchers from UCLA found that 75 percent of heart attack patients did not present with so-called high-risk cholesterol levels, rather than reevaluating whether the numbers mean jack squat, they theorized that the risk ceiling should be lowered *again* so these oh-so-confusing cases could be lumped into the "at risk" category and be eligible for all associated honors and benefits—like profitable prescription drugs.

Cholesterol "science" in a nutshell: If the shoe doesn't fit, take a few inches off the toes. Then report back to Big Pharma. Did I mention that one of the UCLA researchers also served as a consultant to several pharmaceutical companies? These consulting arrangements may be common, but it doesn't mean that we should gloss over the relationship

Chapter 1. Fat

when evidence warrants a potential change in how or why drugs are prescribed.

For many folks, a single cholesterol reading is nothing but a snapshot of one moment in time anyway. If we believe the conventional wisdom, we'll agonize over one high cholesterol reading. If we believe books like this one, we'll be concerned over a low cholesterol reading. But here's the truth: For better or worse, neither a high nor a low cholesterol reading defines your overall, long-term state of health.

Think about that mortifying photo of you on Facebook. Maybe you're making a hideous face. Maybe you're bug-eyed and rocking six extra chins due to the effects of a few tequila shots. Is that photo representative of your entire life? Or even your entire day? Unless you're pledging a fraternity, it shouldn't be.

Point is: One snapshot doesn't truly define you. (Thank goodness.)

That said, does Photoshopping the bejesus out of that embarrassing photo change the fact that you lip-synced "Like a Prayer" during the wet T-shirt contest at Carlos O'Charlie's? Not a chance. By the same token, it's totally ridiculous to artificially manipulate your cholesterol numbers (read: take medication to change them) rather than own them, learn from them as you are right now, and watch them over time to identify potential patterns for the sake of self-knowledge.

Overall, what we need to know is this: The numbers really don't tell us what we've been trained to think they do. High cholesterol isn't necessarily bad, and low cholesterol isn't necessarily good. If we do some digging, we can find scientific studies evaluating trends and risk factors over time that factor in multiple tests and individual data, whose results indicate that chronically low cholesterol may be a red flag and that chronically high cholesterol is far less risky than we once thought. We'll talk about that, but remember the point: We need to question what we've been taught. We might need to ask ourselves a few questions that actually do paint a picture of our health: How often do I get sick? How quickly do I recover? How are my stress levels? And how the heck do I feel?

Maybe the truth is that there is no clear "perfect number" for any given moment, because each of our lives is fundamentally different. Cholesterol in the blood just is what it is, and a person's need (yes, it's a need) for more or less cholesterol can change based on the answers to those questions. It can also change based on time of day, physical state, stress, thyroid function, and simple individual variation.

It's time to reevaluate what high cholesterol means to us. It's time to acknowledge that high cholesterol does not absolutely spell heart disease or death.

What is it good for? Absolutely everything!

Cholesterol is classified as a lipid—a fat—but it's actually a waxy steroid. No, not the kind that gets Major League Baseball's britches in a twist. This steroid is an organic compound that serves as the building block for cell structures and hormones, including sex hormones (hubba hubba). Your body uses it to make bile and vitamin D, and it plays a major role in serotonin production and brain function. It's also a powerful antioxidant.

So you'd be right to deduce that cholesterol helps us stay randy, well-nourished, smart, happy, and healthy at the most fundamental level. Without cholesterol, our cell membranes would become weak and floppy. Think of it like Jenga—pull out too much of the structure, and the whole thing comes crashing down.

Blood cholesterol and cholesterol-rich foods are major players in our resistance to infection, both directly and indirectly. Blood cholesterol can disable toxins produced by bacteria and support the immune system as it fights infection. Long before we developed antibiotics, a blend of cholesterol-rich raw egg yolks and cream was often used to "cure" tuberculosis. Why? Because cholesterol-rich foods like this are some of the most nutrient-dense foods on the planet, supplying critical nutrients like vitamin A, vitamin D, choline, and arachidonic acid, which are vital for bolstering the immune system. Incidentally, I haven't been sick since I—figuratively speaking—dived headfirst into a vat of hollandaise sauce.

Cholesterol's health-enhancing powers even apply to some gnarly medical problems. According to Campbell-McBride:

> *LDL cholesterol, or so-called bad cholesterol, directly binds [to] and inactivates dangerous bacterial toxins. . . . One of the most lethal toxins is produced by a widely spread bacterium,* Staphylococcus aureus, *which is the cause of MRSA, a common hospital infection. This toxin can literally dissolve red blood cells. However, it does not work in the presence of LDL cholesterol.*

And it's not just our immune system that is weakened without cholesterol. Our hormone levels are jeopardized (low testosterone, dudes?) when we remove the raw materials we need to create them, and studies show that people with a long history of low cholesterol have a higher risk of cancer.

Remember how I said cholesterol plays a major part in brain function? Without cholesterol, folks may be more prone to memory loss—a known side effect of statin use—as discovered by a former NASA scientist and astronaut, Duane Graveline, whose own experience with statins prompted him to write *Lipitor: Thief of Memory.* Cholesterol is the key player in brain synapse formation, and synapses are the orchestrators of our ability to learn and remember, two faculties that truly enable us to function in the world.

Beyond that, low cholesterol has been observed in individuals with suicidal tendencies and those who have committed violent crimes. The evidence is so strong, in fact, that a leading researcher on low cholesterol and statin drugs has determined the relationship between low cholesterol and violent behavior to be causal. In other words, low cholesterol isn't "associated with" or "correlated to" violent behavior—it can actually *cause* violent behavior.

But wait. Cholesterol—especially high cholesterol—is supposed to be *dangerous,* right? It causes heart disease, after all. Doesn't it?

No!

When something—high-fiber cereal, for instance, or a statin drug—is said to "help lower cholesterol," we assume this means it'll prevent heart disease. The "lower cholesterol equals less heart disease" idea has been accepted and regurgitated ad nauseam. And it makes me want to "ad nauseam" all over my three-egg omelet.

Here's the problem: Cholesterol doesn't *cause* heart disease in the first place. So concluding that lowering cholesterol is the best way to prevent heart disease makes a total, complete, utter boner out of science.

The notion that cholesterol causes heart disease has been abandoned by many physicians and scientists. Why? Because after decades of studies and spin, there's still no hard evidence to prove the hypothesis.

Suddenly, spending my hard-earned money (or insurance coverage) on a cholesterol-lowering drug that has little to give but side effects and a false sense of security sounds less appealing. I could spin my wheels at far more enjoyable tasks, like trying to make sense of *Twilight.*

What's really going on under the hood?

Let's go a bit deeper by looking at so-called good (HDL) cholesterol and bad (LDL) cholesterol. LDL and HDL are lipoproteins, particles that carry cholesterol. These lipoproteins are composed of other materials as well, such as polyunsaturated fats, which, when damaged, probably *do* play a direct role in heart disease.

As we've already learned, LDL cholesterol (that is, choles-terol carried by low-density lipoproteins) can protect us from nasty infections, so why do we think it's bad?

When there's a problem in the body that requires healing, cholesterol is part of the healing response. LDL takes cho-lesterol to the site of the damage; HDL takes it away. If we posit that LDL is bad simply because it's brought to the site of a problem, we may as well, as Campbell-McBride puts it, call an ambulance on its way to an accident a "bad ambu-lance" and an ambulance on its way to the hospital a "good ambulance."

Here's the deal: When injury or illness occurs in your body, an inflammatory response is dispatched to deal with the problem so that the injury can heal. This applies to any tissue, not just the heart.

Imagine you really, really suck in the kitchen. You're get-ting ready to use your immersion blender to whip up some apple–butternut squash bisque. You notice just a moment be-fore you blend that something is stuck to the blade. So, as your right hand pushes the "on" button, your left reaches in to clear the debris. Finger slice city. (True story, unfortunately.)

To heal the damage your gawd-awful kitchen skills have caused, your body initiates what's called an *inflammatory response*. The area reddens, throbs, scabs over, and finally heals.

Yep, inflammation is actually a good thing. Without it, no damage would ever heal. But could your finger ever fully mend if you kept slicing it open, creating a constant storm of never-ending irritation and unsuccessful repair?

Not a chance. Our bodies are able to handle individual stressors, but chronic, repeated ones? Not so much. Like *Jersey Shore* spin-offs, eventually it all gets to be too much.

So it is with the chronic insults from lifestyle factors—smoking, too much sugar or too few nutrients, chronic stress—and their resulting health problems, including free-radical damage, infection, high blood pressure, and chronically elevated blood sugar and insulin. These problems set the stage for damage to the arterial walls, leading to inflammation that's intended to repair the issue. Add damaged LDL—a consequence of damaged polyunsaturated fat intake, likely from crop oils—which stimulates an endless loop of scratch-and-patch within the body, and you've got an ongoing problem of well-intentioned inflammation that's never able to do its job.

So when we talk about "clogged arteries" in the context of heart disease, we're mostly talking about inflammation gone wild, an inflammatory response to irritation within the body that is never able to resolve. The materials that converge on the site are known as *plaque* or *arterial plaque,* and this is what actually makes a "clogged artery." This doesn't happen just to the cardiovascular system, but we tend to focus on the heart simply because the heart is particularly vulnerable due to the nature of its responsibilities. It's kind of a big deal.

Picture putting caulk in a crack (I know, there's no way to keep from giggling at that phrase). You patch the gap and then stop caulking. You've made your repair—good as new. Now, imagine you never stop patching. The caulk overflows the crack and piles up, creating a big ugly mess. Stuff ends up where it doesn't belong.

So it is with the inflammatory response and all the healing substances, from cholesterol to collagen, that attempt to fix things that just won't stop breaking. The process of constant inflammation and unsuccessful repair means that they pile up where we don't want them. Plaque is the result of a lesion that develops in the messy muck of a chronic, out-of-control inflammatory response. And why we see cholesterol there? Because any attempt at healing—successful or not—means that the body has to build new cells.

Cells are made of fats and cholesterol. Unfortunately, we can't change that, and replacing fats in the diet with more "whole grain" won't build healthier "whole-grain" cells. Fats and cholesterol are the building blocks for life. We must learn to love 'em.

So the plaque buildup process has nothing to do with some evil plot perpetrated by cholesterol lurking in our egg yolks or our bloodstreams, packing itself into our arteries and causing us to croak. Cholesterol is a very different animal (pun intended) from what we've been led to believe.

Your cholesterol level doesn't predict your propensity for plaque, either. In a study of cardiovascular tissue from more than 22,000 autopsies performed in fourteen different nations, researchers found no difference in plaque formation between those with low cholesterol and those with high cholesterol. People with low cholesterol were prone to just as much blockage as those with high cholesterol.

As Ellison states, "There is no correlation or relationship between low cholesterol and the [slowing or stopping of] . . . atherosclerosis—the number one cause of heart disease."

This is me beating a dead horse: Lower cholesterol doesn't prevent heart disease. Because cholesterol doesn't cause heart disease.

In fact, according to Ellison, so-called low cholesterol has been associated with "worse outcomes in heart failure patients and impaired survival, while high cholesterol improved survival rates. . . . Findings showed that elevated cholesterol among patients was not associated with hypertension, diabetes, or coronary heart disease."

Your blood cholesterol is managed by your body in response to what's going on inside and out. Your cholesterol may rise based on what you probably already know is happening: Systemic stress. Crappy diet or lifestyle choices. Thyroid issues. Any health problem. Healing from surgery or a dental procedure. The process of rebalancing the body after weight loss. Recovery from competition. Injuries sustained from banging your head against the wall. (Do you know the feeling?)

Cholesterol levels also rise naturally as we get older, and for good reason. As our bodies go through the aging process, they simply need more healing support and fortification. Cholesterol provides this. Botox, unfortunately, does not.

In these cases, we can consider cholesterol a marker or even a messenger that's telling you, *I'm here for you.*

If you have a healthy, active lifestyle; if you manage stress conscientiously and have a smidgen of self-awareness; and if your focus is on real, whole, nutrient-dense foods, your cholesterol is probably exactly where it needs to be. Your inflammatory process likely works as it should, and the potential for dysfunction is low.

If, on the other hand, you follow more of a standard American diet-stress-crash-repeat lifestyle, you need to fix the problem, whether or not you have high cholesterol.

In other words: Cholesterol isn't the freaking problem.

So *why* would I want to take statins?

"The cholesterol-lowering myth being spread by pharmaceutical companies worldwide," Ellison says, "could rightfully be considered the deadliest health myth in the history of mankind." Bold statement. Could it be true?

When we artificially lower cholesterol with drugs, we can cripple the body's ability to function naturally, to build new cells and do everything else it needs to do to keep us well.

As I'll discuss in upcoming chapters, plants and fungi have defense mechanisms to protect them from predators. Where we have arms to punch and legs to run, plants and fungi have poisons and toxins. The fungus from which statins are derived—red yeast rice—uses a defense that cripples cholesterol production, but it also cripples production of co-enzyme Q10 (CoQ10), an antioxidant produced by the body that is present in every single cell and that is critical for energy production in heart cells.

This plant defense mechanism is designed to cause damage to a predator. I'm not so sure about using it to treat a not-so-problematic "problem," especially when it relates to something as important as, ya know, the heart.

But considering that the imaginary "problem" with cholesterol was dreamed up and disseminated by the very folks who make foods that they say solve it and the drugs that they say treat it, I suppose it all makes sense.

In an evil, twisted, lose-hope-in-humanity kind of way.

Statins are sometimes praised for their anti-inflammatory properties, which are independent of their cholesterol-lowering properties. Fortunate accident? I suppose, but it sure comes with a long warning label. And guess what's guaranteed to be a side-effect-free, non-CoQ10-depleting, drug-free, idiot-proof inflammation buster? An anti-inflammatory diet and lifestyle! And what comprises an anti-inflammatory diet and lifestyle? The very recommendations I make throughout this book!

A few thousand words later, can we put a bow on this cholesterol thing?

So we understand that cholesterol isn't the demon it's made out to be, that it does not cause heart disease, and that lowering dietary or blood cholesterol has not been shown to keep heart disease at bay. So what's the ultimate conclusion?

Eat Egg Beaters and put statins in the drinking water? Not even close.

Cholesterol in real, natural, whole foods is not to be feared. Neither is high blood cholesterol. Eat egg yolks with abandon—they are a health food. Why? Because the cholesterol in real food, like egg yolks, is not just a powerful antioxidant. It's also packaged with other nutrients we need.

Neither the cholesterol in our food nor the cholesterol in our blood causes heart disease, and when it comes to the cholesterol in our blood, remember that it's there for a reason. It's a healing substance. Blood cholesterol numbers alone mean less than a third-place ribbon at a potato sack race, because what really matters is your overall state of health. If you're stressed, experiencing systemic inflammation, and eating lots of crop oils that contribute to damaged LDL, you likely need some help with your entire diet and lifestyle. Whacking blindly at your cholesterol readings with statins that may do more harm than good? Likely not the solution.

Final answer: Don't fear cholesterol, and don't fear real food!

This also goes for another favorite: savory, satisfying saturated fat.

Saturated science? Fat chance

We've talked about the powerful interests behind the nutritional developments of the last fifty years. We've done our hand-wringing over dietary and blood cholesterol. But what about the so-called science surrounding our aversion to saturated fat? Did it ever pan out?

Not at all. Even if we set aside the vital roles fat plays in the body, there's a glaring lack of evidence against natural saturated fat. An analysis in the *American Journal of Clinical Nutrition* evaluated more than twenty studies with a combined pool of nearly 350,000 subjects for proof of a connection between saturated fat and heart disease. The investigation found that there was "no significant evidence for concluding that dietary saturated fat is associated with an increased risk [of heart disease]."

What about that old run-on phrase *arterycloggingsaturatedfat*? Turns out it's weak sauce. A study in the *Lancet* found no association between how much saturated fat we eat and the amount of arterial plaque we develop. This means that eating saturated fat doesn't send that fat straight to the arteries. Again, arterial plaque is the consequence of chronic inflammation run wild, not steak night. Unlike pantyhose and Canada geese, saturated fat doesn't migrate to places it's not welcome. Good news for steak lovers: That cow stays right where it belongs. In your belly.

So why all the drama? The line between the overall demonization of fat and the exclusive targeting of saturated fat can seem blurry at times, but insofar as the two ideas resulted in a bevy of "fat-free" and "low-fat" packaged foods, they certainly deserve united credit for the bass-ackwards nutrition information and so-called healthy foods most of us grew up with.

Saturated fat was demonized in the first place because we thought it raised cholesterol, which freaked us out because we'd been told that higher cholesterol led to heart disease. At some point, we stopped caring about the whole proposed chain of events—false as it is—and decided that saturated fat "clogged arteries" too, as if the human body were just a big jumble of copper plumbing and any type of fat or cholesterol would plug us up.

But if cholesterol doesn't cause heart disease, and if saturated fat doesn't jam up the arteries like a clump of leaves in a storm drain, then we don't give a hoot whether natural saturated fats raise cholesterol or not. *Amiright?*

It's worth noting, though, just for the sake of further decimating these old myths, that certain natural saturated fats have been shown to raise "good" cholesterol, and many studies indicating that they raise "bad" cholesterol are simply poorly constructed or interpreted. Most important, there is no predetermined cholesterol outcome when you eat saturated fat. Higher cholesterol can decrease with the consumption of almost any fat, including saturated fat; and low cholesterol can increase with the consumption of most fats as well.

What does this mean? It means that our biology is beautifully individualized and our bodies aren't machines with a predetermined output for every input, but dynamic organisms, navigating and negotiating our unique personal landscapes with an innate logic that exists whether a team of pharmaceutical researchers have studied it or not. Human experiences, like fats, are as diverse as the reality television shows recorded on my DVR.

However, keep in mind that the idea that saturated fat raises cholesterol, thereby causing heart disease, is a myth. Other studies linking animal fat to colon and breast cancer have been interpreted so poorly, says Masterjohn, that upon further investigation, it's crop oils that correlate with cancer.

Considering that margarine and shortening are generally blends of crop oils—for a long stretch of history, partially hydrogenated ones—and usually include additives like emulsifiers; and considering that butter from pastured cows actually contains cancer-fighting nutrients like conjugated linoleic acid, I'll just stick with the real thing.

So here's where I'm driving this boat: Natural saturated fat is not just better for you than anything the crop oil industry has ever created, it's flat-out spectacular. It's even more amazing than beating your husband in Virtual Scrabble because the word *za* is in the online dictionary.

It's amazing for health reasons, which I'll discuss momentarily; and it's amazing for its taste and versatility. Unlike flavorless, deodorized, highly refined oils, natural saturated fats impart *flavor*. Life simply isn't complete without the complex, rich flavors of butter, clarified butter, ghee, a good cut of steak, coconut oil, home-rendered lard, schmaltz, tallow, and—yes—even cocoa butter.

Do a few of those sound weird or unfamiliar to you? Fifty years ago, many of them were kitchen staples. Before the technology for extracting oils from soybeans, corn, and canola became commonplace and ridiculously profitable, the most readily available fats in the United States were saturated animal fats. These fats occur naturally and require no factory intervention.

Making lard, in fact, is almost easier than the effort it takes to drive to the store, pick up some crop oil, and, ten years later, undergo medical treatment for the plethora of health issues associated with long-term use of highly processed fats.

We aren't the only country that once made heavy use of saturated fats. Some countries never gave up the practice. What we now call the "French paradox"—the curious fact that the French eat plenty of saturated fat yet suffer low incidence of heart disease—is actually the "Eskimo-Chinese-Greek-Puerto Rican-Okinawan-and-beyond paradox."

People in cultures across the planet, even those commonly labeled as vegetarian by unscrupulous researchers, consume saturated fat and cholesterol-rich foods and live in excellent health. Absolutely no "paradoxical" culture consumes processed crop oils in the types and amounts we Americans do today.

It's not whether a fat is saturated, plant-derived, or animal-based that we should be worried about anyway. Here are the three things we *actually* need to think about when we choose fats: First, how processed is it? Second, how stable is it? And, third, how many nutrients come with it? (The fourth criterion—How tasty is it?—didn't make the cut. It gave animal fat an unfair advantage.)

Can you guess which fats are the most processed, the most highly refined, and the least healthy?

Margarine. Soybean oil. Canola oil. Corn oil. Cottonseed oil. Trans fats. These highly processed plant-based fats are often referred to as *vegetable oils,* even though they're *not from freaking vegetables*. Soybean oil and corn oil are particularly rich in polyunsaturated fat, and canola and cottonseed oil contain their fair share as well.

So if natural saturated fats aren't the villains we once thought, what is it that makes them special? How are animal fats different from crop oils? And what is it about fat that offends our delicate, diet-conscious sensibilities?

Your fat: How processed is it?

The less processing a fat requires to make it to our tables, the better. The intensive refinement process that crop oils require is downright horrifying, from the frightening mechanics of it to the way the whole process destroys what few nutrients are there in the first place.

We could never in a million years make these crop oils at home, because producing them requires a highly specialized, technology-driven, factory-based refining process. Seeds of these crops are often subject to processing before they're even planted in the form of genetic modification, which is just another facet of the processed-food industry. This technology has been applied to 93 percent of soybeans, 88 percent of corn, 94 percent of cottonseed, and 90 percent of canola crops in the United States. The genetic modification process was developed not so we could "feed the world," as propaganda suggests, but for the sheer profitability of manipulating plant DNA to create higher-yield, herbicide-resistant plants that have never existed, and could never exist, naturally in a balanced ecosystem.

While hybridization and selective breeding of plants has occurred for centuries within regional foodsheds, this natural process is one carried out by hand—or sometimes by bees, which, ironically, are being decimated by pesticides used by the same corporations behind the genetic modification of crops. Natural hybridization is distinct from genetic modification in every way. Says Wenonah Hauter in *Foodopoly,* "It is different than the traditional selective breeding of plants over many generations. . . . At this time, splicing genes is a very expensive business that requires state-of-the-art laboratories and highly paid scientists."

The consequences of hijacking nature for corporate gain are clear: Genetically modified foods have been blamed for the development of pesticide-resistant weeds and pests and are a subject of constant debate for their potential impact on human and environmental health.

Once these crops, whether genetically modified or not, are harvested, they go through another round of industrial beat-downs. Oils from corn, soy, cotton, and canola crops are extracted through a chemical-filled, high-heat process, followed by a process of deodorization and further refinement to remove odor and impurities. The process of getting soy oil from soy, for example, requires solvent extraction, degumming, bleaching, and deodorization, followed by more processing to keep the rancidity-prone oil from spoiling before it leaves the factory. It's no surprise that, until the 1940s, this oil was thought to be unsuitable for human consumption but appropriate for use as a paint additive.

These damaging processes yield a profitable product, not a healthy one, and the true driving force is the commodity crop industry—not the health industry.

The more processing applied to these crops, the more profitable they become. Oil is just a by-product of the profit machine. Ninety-eight percent of soy grown in the United States goes to factory-farmed animal feed. The other by-products are sold off as candle wax or various food additives; soy lecithin, once called "lecithin sludge," finds its way into everything from chocolate to baby formula. By-products of corn production are used as thickeners, like cornstarch, and sweeteners, like high-fructose corn syrup. Canola by-product is sold as animal feed. Cottonseed oil is a by-product of the cotton industry.

Processing, processing, processing means profits, profits, profits.

We often think of "nothing going to waste" as a good thing, and it is in theory. However, the point is lost when every smidge of the original product requires a factory, industrial chemicals, plastic packaging, teams of scientists and engineers, and artificial fertilizers, as industrial crops do.

Crop oil processing is also environmentally unsound. When it comes to the refining of soy oil, for example, according to research chemist KeShun Liu, the waste products of production can pose dangers to the environment when not properly contained and disposed. For this reason, "wastewater control, solid waste disposal, and air pollution control" are requisite co-industries.

By contrast, we can make use of the entire animal and every nourishing part—no factory needed, no nonbiodegradable plastic packaging, no chemical extraction, no environmentally dangerous by-products. The same pasture-raised pig that gives us pork chops can also give us lard for cooking and soap, pork belly for bacon, blood for pudding and sausage, and bones for mineral-rich homemade broth. That's truly making good use of every part of the animal, in a way that's better for us and for the environment, and that provides a better life for the animal itself. And that's how it used to work.

So far, crop oils don't stand up to scrutiny, and it's not just because they're more processed than my hair color in high school. With this kind of intensive processing, we can only imagine the type of beat-down the nutritional value takes— that is, if there's any nutritional value in crop oils at all.

Let's remember our food roots: We're programmed to eat fat and cholesterol as humans have for thousands of years, in their least-processed forms, within their natural packaging (meaning animal products, whole seafood, egg yolks, avocados, coconuts, nuts, and olives) or after they've been extracted using extremely light, traditional, factory-not-required methods that preserve their built-in structure, antioxidant content, and nutrient density. We see this with unrefined coconut oil, cold-pressed olive and sesame oils, and animal fats such as lard, tallow, butter, clarified butter, and ghee.

Many healthy fats from unrefined plants and properly raised creatures come with even more built-in protection that helps preserve the antioxidants and nutrients that make them so valuable in the first place. This protective packaging is the food itself. Coconut oil comes packaged in the coconut, animal fat comes packaged in a juicy steak, and fish oils come with the fish. We could grow or raise and render these fats ourselves if we wanted to, as people did for hundreds of years using only the supplies they had on hand. The same cannot be said of crop oils.

Though we often choose to allow a middleman to do the growing, raising, and rendering for us when it comes to those less-processed fats, that's certainly not required. However, the less responsibility we take for our own personal food supply, the wealthier the processed-food industry becomes—and the less healthy we become.

Our health is a product of our nutrition, and highly refined crop oils have several nutrition-related issues, the first of which is nutrient destruction and loss.

When fats, especially those from crops, are isolated into oils through a long refinement process, each step of that process makes the oils more vulnerable to nutrition degradation and damage. Of the relatively few nutrients in crop oils, most are lost during refinement. Vitamin E, for example—an antioxidant found in soybeans—is lost during the deodorization process. Carotenes and chlorophyll, often touted as healthy plant constituents, are also lost during crop oil refining.

But this isn't even the most frightening nutritional problem. It's what happens to the fats themselves, and what they can do to our bodies, when the antioxidants are gone.

Your fat: How stable is it?

Stability isn't just something we should look for in a mate. It's also critical when it comes to the fats we eat.

Crop oils are, by nature, unstable. When I talk about stability, I'm talking about one simple concept: the ability to resist oxidative damage. There are a few other words for oxidative damage—lipid peroxidation, auto-oxidation, oxidative stress, free-radical damage, rancidification—but they all mean the same thing. Weaknesses in the bonds of the vulnerable fatty acids, called *unsaturated bonds,* react with oxygen, especially in the absence of critical antioxidants. Like a piece of metal rusting, this reaction initiates a process of progressive degeneration, and the fat continues to break down. Damaged, oxidized, warped fatty acids from the unstable oils we eat are incorporated into our own cells, and these fats and their by-products are implicated in premature aging, cancer, heart disease, and even damage to our very DNA.

It comes as no surprise that the more processed a fat is, the more unstable it is. Once the crop oil refinement process is complete and any potentially protective antioxidants are gone, there's nothing left but a fragile, stripped-down, damaged oil that's vulnerable to even more damage.

The vast majority of highly processed fats start out at a stability disadvantage, even before their antioxidants are destroyed and they're factory-freaked into oblivion. That's because most highly processed fats are of the predominantly polyunsaturated variety. (Elsewhere, you may see polyunsaturated fatty acid abbreviated as PUFA, monounsaturated as MUFA, and saturated as SFA.)

Polyunsaturated fats are, by nature, extremely fragile and thus vulnerable to damage. Remember, polyunsaturated fats have two or more unsecured links in their fatty acid chains, and when they're refined and exposed to insults like heat, industrial chemicals, and oxygen—as crop oils are in the extraction and refinement process—they've got absolutely nothing protecting those unsecured links. Free radicals, which come along with those insults, plug into the chains and cause oxidative damage.

So polyunsaturated fats are unstable to begin with, and the process used to extract them only compounds the problem: The more heat, light, air, chemicals, and overall abuse needed to pull the fats from their natural packaging, the more oxidative damage these fats incur.

Of course, we want to avoid oxidative damage and all its cellular consequences. Unfortunately, it's tough to fight oxidative damage when we stack the cards against ourselves by eating oils that are chock-full of it. No amount of antioxidants will make up for the dangers that highly processed oils pose to our bodies—we could eat a whole bush of antioxidant-rich blueberries and it wouldn't come close to stopping the oxidative damage caused by the broke-ass polyunsaturated fats in our kitchen cabinets.

Yet polyunsaturated fats from crop oils are the fats that many doctors and health professionals tell us to eat in place of more stable options, like animal fat!

Why? I'll tell ya why: because they've been snowed, just as we once were. They've been taught the same old fear of animal fats, based on the same old misconception that all animal fats are saturated fats and the same old false belief that saturated fats and cholesterol cause heart disease, all of which are based on the same old misinformation we've already put to rest.

Despite all this polyunsaturated doom-and-gloom, there are two highly beneficial types of polyunsaturated fats that, unlike crop oils, are very important to the human body. These are the omega fats: an omega-6 fat known as arachidonic acid and an omega-3 fat known as DHA (often referred to in supplements as "fish oil" simply because it's found in abundance in fish). These fats keep the process of inflammation in balance and offer a slew of other benefits that I'll discuss further in chapter 4.

Fortunately, we don't need crop oils to obtain these omega fats. We can get sufficient arachidonic acid from whole, unprocessed animal foods like egg yolks, and we can get sufficient DHA from oily, whole fish. That emphasis on "whole" is important: Despite the ever-popular practice of isolating fish oil from the fish it naturally comes in, these are the same polyunsaturates that are vulnerable to damage when extracted or refined from their natural sources. Extracting the oil from fish can damage these fragile fats. That's why we should get them by eating fish, not from the fish oil pill industry—which, incidentally, much like the crop oil industry, sells its protein-rich fish meal as animal feed.

Seems there's always an ulterior motive when it comes to processing polyunsaturates.

The good fats I'm fighting for—fats from properly raised animals, sustainably caught whole seafood, coconuts, olives, avocados, and nuts—are fully edible in their natural vehicles. Some of them are easily extracted through the safe process of pressing or home-rendering. People have been doing that for hundreds, even thousands, of years.

The natural, healthy fats that we're meant to eat are inherently stable by virtue of their higher saturation, the vehicles they come in, or the nutrients they're packaged with. Or, in some cases, all three.

The highly saturated fats from properly raised animals are more stable not just because they are more saturated but also because the animals themselves are naturally fortified with antioxidant nutrients, such as cholesterol and vitamin A. Seafood, which contains vulnerable but healthful polyunsaturated omega-3 fats, has natural packaging (it's called the fish) that protects those fats from damage.

Olives and olive oil come packaged with antioxidant polyphenols. Coconut oil is so highly saturated that it's extremely unlikely to oxidize. Nuts, which contain both monounsaturated and polyunsaturated fats, protect those fats within the nut itself, so they're less likely to oxidize.

Lightly pressing a fruit or nut—as Mediterranean cultures have done with olives for thousands of years, Asian cultures have done with sesame, and tropical cultures have done with palm and coconut—yields a stable, healthy fat.

Getting the picture?

When natural, antioxidant-rich fats are used for cooking, their stability is better preserved because of the antioxidants they're fortified with naturally. Extremely saturated fats, like those from coconuts and clarified butter, are stable by virtue of their saturation.

When antioxidant-poor, highly processed, less-saturated fats, like those from crop oils, are exposed to heat from cooking, they sustain even more damage than the factory-freaking process already caused. Damage on top of damage: Two wrongs *don't* make a right.

In other words: Factory-freaked, processed, polyunsaturated fats *bad*. Naturally occurring, minimally processed saturated fats *good*.

And what about monounsaturated fats? These fats, contrary to popular belief, aren't found only in plants (although they are present in olives, avocados, and nuts). We also find monounsaturated fats in lard, butter, and other animal fats. These fats are made even more stable by the other fats they're packaged with: Monounsaturated fat packaged with saturated fat (as in butter, tallow, or lard) is far more stable than monounsaturated fat without saturated fat (as in canola oil).

Monounsaturated fat from unprocessed plant sources—such as whole olives, cold-pressed olive oil, avocados, and nuts—is less stable than more highly saturated fats but far more stable than processed polyunsaturated fat from margarine, corn, canola, cottonseed, and soy, not because they're packaged with saturated fat but because they're packaged with natural protection: the plant itself, or at least the antioxidants that come with it.

That brings us to the final judge of a fat's worthiness: its nutrient density.

Your fat: How many nutrients come with it?

Nutrient density may be the single most important factor that sets fats from properly raised animals apart from even the most unprocessed, stable plant oils. This is why animal fats are so important.

While plants like olives and avocados certainly come packaged with nutrients, they're not the same nutrients that we find in living creatures. I wish they were. It wasn't easy for me to come to terms with my biological place in—or my responsibility to—the food chain.

The fat-phobic hysteria of the last few decades has driven us to forget that the most important nutrients we can possibly get are all housed with fats. These are called fat-soluble vitamins because—duh—our bodies need fat to absorb them. Mother Nature strikes again!

And not just any fat is needed to make use of critical nutrients. Masterjohn states that fats lower in polyunsaturated fat appear to "provide the best absorption of fat-soluble nutrients. When compared to corn oil, for example, olive oil roughly doubles the absorption of [the nutrients] lycopene and astaxanthin in rats." It appears, then, that the more saturated the fat, the more it helps us absorb certain nutrients. Which makes sense, because fat-soluble nutrients are generally packaged that way anyway.

Animal fats are dense in fat-soluble vitamins A, D, and K_2, which are critical to human health. Contrary to popular belief, we do *not* get these vitamins from plants.

Not to worry, though, because plant-eating animals raised in their natural environments use their unique digestive machinery to turn vitamin building blocks into their active, fat-soluble forms, and they store these active forms in their tissue. We get vitamins A, D, and K_2 by eating those animals.

Fat-soluble vitamins play a role in eye health, bone health, heart health, skin health, reproductive health, immune system health, lung health, and emotional health. So . . . yeah. They're kind of a big deal.

Lard is rich in vitamin D, as are oily fish like salmon and sardines. Red meat is dense in vitamin A. Liver and egg yolks are rich in vitamins A and K_2. Animals also offer us extremely bioavailable minerals and other nutrients like conjugated linoleic acid, which may help fight cancer. A thoughtful omnivore will get the entire spectrum of fat-soluble nutrients through respectful nose-to-tail creature-eating.

Crop oils are rich in . . . baggage, like easily damaged, highly processed polyunsaturated fat. (What losers, right?)

High-fat dairy products like butter, clarified butter, and ghee from animals raised in their natural environments with their natural diets are incredibly stable, concentrated sources of fat-soluble vitamins. They've been highly prized for centuries by healthy cultures around the world, and science backs up this ancestral wisdom: An Australian study found that higher dairy fat consumption resulted in a 69 percent lower risk for cardiovascular death. Those who ate no dairy or exclusively low-fat dairy were three times more likely to die from heart disease or stroke.

Speaking of the virtues of full-fat dairy, like butter, brings me to the world's greatest nutritional scourge: butter substitutes.

Margarine:
The nightmare on Butter Boulevard

Margarine is the greatest culinary and dietary atrocity ever to be inflicted upon our society. It's the perfect example of the ridiculous road our fear of real food has taken us down. It's a saturated-fat-phobic butter-phile's dream. Its texture and color remind us of the real thing, but its marketing—and its ingredients list—reminds us that it's anything but.

Yet that's not how margarine began. Margarine, in fact, was born of a butter shortage.

In 1869, a French chemist named Hippolyte Mège Mouriès (sounds like *margarine*) was charged with creating a product that could take the place of butter in both texture and nutrient density.

At the time, regional drought in Europe had made cows unable to produce milk with enough fat content that it could be turned into butter. The food supply then was—as it naturally is—dependent on the weather. No rain meant no grass, and no grass meant the cows were starving. There was no butter.

Knowing how important energy-dense and nutrient-rich butter was to the vast working class, a butter-replacement project was commissioned, possibly by Napoleon III himself. The intent was to improve the nutrition available to lower-income families who couldn't afford enough calorie-filled fat to thrive.

Mège believed that the replacement fat had to be beef-derived, so he created a mixture of beef fat and skim milk. It worked. It was a sufficient replacement for butter during those hard times.

For a long time, butter remained a rich man's food and the beef-fat-based margarine a poor man's nutrition substitute. But as the industry grew and the partial hydrogenation process was developed near the turn of the twentieth century, the margarine industry was able to grow by shifting away from animal fats and focusing on crop oils.

The partial hydrogenation process enabled—and continues to enable—crop oils to be turned into solid fats. Until the technology was developed for extracting oils from domestic crops like corn, canola, and soybeans, faraway countries supplied coconut and palm oil for partial hydrogenation. This set the stage for a global trade in raw materials for margarine production, which meant that this fabulous product (sarcasm) now had global reach.

Remember, the doubling of margarine production from 1920 to 1950, along with the use of partially hydrogenated oils beginning around 1900, happens to coincide with the rise of heart disease as a public health concern in the United States. Just sayin'.

Regardless of the fats used, the partial hydrogenation process generates trans fats, and for many years partial hydrogenation was the only way to make margarines and shortening. Today, some butter substitutes are made through the use of emulsifiers—also by-products of crop oil production—to thicken them without trans fats. Until the 1950s, however, we didn't know that the trans fats created by partial hydrogenation were bad. We just knew that turning oils into solids meant never having to rely on the fickle supply of animal fat again.

As agricultural oil production grew around the world beginning around 1900, creating the beginnings of the global oil-trade economy, we suddenly had a new conundrum: what to do with all the protein-rich meal left over from the crops (including soybean and cottonseed) that were used for margarine oil?

Great Scott! We'll feed it to the animals! Yes, the ever-growing margarine market played a direct role the development of the factory-farming industry from approximately 1920 to today.

Agricultural oil production is, and always has been, about industry. It was never about health.

But what about the *calories*, yo!

So let's get truthful about our fear of natural fat. If we can dismiss fears about its chemical structure or cardiovascular effects, what else is there to be afraid of?

Simple: calories.

But we've been obsessed with calories for so long that we've forgotten what's supposed to come *with* our calories: nutrients. And the fact that fats have more calories per gram (nine, compared to four from proteins and carbs) isn't necessarily a bad thing. More calories per gram means more energy per bite. It means you can feel full having eaten less.

At one time, when Big Business wasn't supplying us with a flood of croppy, crappy, cheap, always-available, nutrient-poor calories, finding food that provided plenty of nutrient-dense energy was actually a good thing. The problem isn't too many calories per nutrient-rich bite. It's too many nutrient-poor bites per person.

When a body is poorly nourished—as it is when we consume damaged oils, a low-fat diet, or a diet high in processed foods (even those commonly considered healthy)—the risk of uncontrolled cravings and continued irrational eating just goes up. When our bodies don't have the nutrients they need—the nutrients from fats—for basic tasks like cellular repair, hormonal function or even damage control, they let us know: Appetite increases, and we're driven to eat more as our bodies seek nutrients from anything, at any cost. That's why diets don't work, especially low-fat diets; they often restrict nourishment along with calories.

But nourishing our bodies with healthy, nutrient-dense fats keeps our cells in good shape. Hormonal signaling, which is critical in appetite regulation, remains balanced. Fat, unlike carbohydrate, is used by the body for many things besides energy. While excess carbohydrates can be converted into fat and stored, healthy fats are used up in a multitude of ways: for nutrient transport, hormone function, cell structure and repair, and energy.

It's time to think of food and nourishment in a new way.

So what to do?

....

Simple: Eat real food.

We're meant to consume natural, nutrient-dense foods without fear of their natural fat or cholesterol content. We're meant to eat them in as near to their natural state as possible (not low-fat or cholesterol-free versions) to preserve the fatty acids within them.

So eat properly raised animals and minimally processed animal products as well as whole, sustainably caught seafood without fearing the fat that comes with them. This includes whole eggs and whole cuts of beef, bison, lamb, poultry, pork, venison, or any other creature raised in its natural environment, eating its natural diet. It's how healthy humans ate for thousands of years.

Eat the fats you know are unprocessed, stable, and nutrient-dense—fats like lard, tallow, suet, and poultry fat from animals raised in their natural environments, eating their natural diets.

Choose stable, traditional plant fats, like coconut and antioxidant-rich olive or sesame oil, and natural, whole plants like avocados, olives, coconuts, and nuts.

Remember that healthy sources of more highly polyunsaturated fats come packaged in their own protective casings, as in nuts and fish. Eat them whole.

Don't eat some of those things. Eat them all, fearlessly and appreciatively.

Chapter 2

....

protein

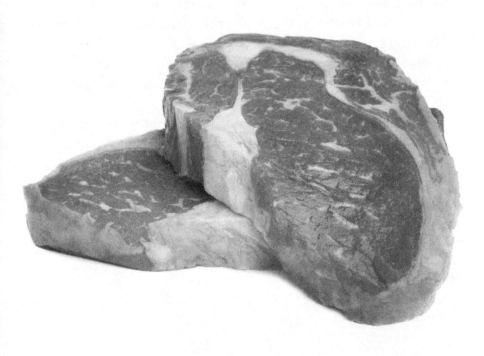

Is killing creatures for food ever okay?

For those of us who choose to eat meat—the flesh of other living, breathing, reproducing, moving, feeling beings—as our primary source of protein, this question hangs in the air over our dinner tables.

As well it should. Something has to die for us to have dinner. That is not a meaningless concept.

At one time, we understood the profound importance of animals to our ability to live well. Now, we're simply confused about where they fit in the eating equation.

Where animals were once an indispensable source of not just nutrient-dense nourishment but also replenishment and stability for the entire homestead, they are now regarded by millions as unwitting victims in a cruel food system that pushes unhealthy, colon-clogging, cancer-causing food on the masses. The more extreme meatless eaters eschew all creature foods—by which I mean meat, eggs, and seafood. Slogans like MEAT IS MURDER decorate T-shirts and protest signs, and trendy books refer to the evils of a "decaying flesh diet." Graphic enough for you?

Our souls, our bodies, and our body fat percentages can only benefit from making the switch to a plants-only diet. Right?

From this convincing pitch have grown countless other just-plants justifications. Veganism is the kind way to eat. Humans can't digest animals. Cow farts cause pollution. We can get sufficient protein from plants.

Here's the truth: Everything we thought we knew about eating creatures, from the way we raise animals to the reasons we avoid meat, is wrong, from top to tail and in more ways than there are Real Housewives. And it's not just the meatless who are off base. Many meat-eaters are also fouling out. (Oh, baseball analogies.) In our constant fiddling with dietary buttons and switches, we've lost the factory default setting, and it's time we all got back to it.

Let's navigate away from the emotional comfort zone, the sound-bite-based diet-food culture, and even indignant carnivory for a while. Let's tell the truth about eating creatures—even though sometimes the truth hurts.

How did we get here? And actually, where the heck are we?

There are several common arguments for eating meat-free these days. These arguments are based on health or compassion, sometimes both. Meat-eaters are often portrayed as ignorant, defiant, skeptical, or simply unapologetic, factory-farming flesh-lovers. But the path that brought us here isn't as clear-cut as good versus bad, kind versus uncaring, or bleeding-heart versus bacon.

Before the interrelated advents of crop oils and animal feedlots, and long before we started worrying—justifiably—about the horrific conditions on factory farms, properly raised, healthy animals played an integral part in the health of the individual, the family, and the land. This includes animals that we domesticated for meat, work, and manure. (Yes, manure. What did we think natural, nonindustrial fertilizers were made of? Poop is important. In a sustainable farming model, animals provide more than just meat.)

Our epic journey from gristle to grains is discussed in more detail in chapter 3, but to summarize several thousand years of dietary changes leading up to our modern misgivings about meat, I'll simply say this: Despite the long-accepted and long-respected roles that wild-hunted or properly raised animals played in human life for thousands of years, both before and after the advent of agriculture, in the early 1900s a few folks began to oppose the eating of animals for reasons vastly different than those we might cite today. These folks were far more concerned about reducing—through vegetarianism, religious devotion, and colon cleansing—the very thing that keeps us, and every other living thing on the planet, from going extinct: our instinct to reproduce.

Kellogg's flaccid flakes

John Harvey Kellogg, who with his brother invented what we now know as cornflakes in 1894, was actually less concerned with cereal than he was with salvation. As a teen, he worked and lived for several years under the tutelage of an extremely religious woman named Ellen White. White believed such vices as "tea, coffee, meat, spices, fashionable dress, and sex" were driving young people to masturbate and thereby become diseased and insane. To live appropriately meant a vegetarian diet and total devotion to fighting the "animal passions."

While I tend to look at human sexuality as a natural part of who we are (it is, after all, how we all got here), influential people in the early part of the twentieth century vehemently disagreed. Their beliefs represented a great departure from the spiritual significance that many native

83

cultures ascribed to the process of hunting, preparing food, and eating.

In 1876, at the age of twenty-four, eighteen years before the accidental discovery of cornflakes, Kellogg took on the role of physician-in-chief at what he would rename the Battle Creek Sanitarium. Although he advocated healthy practices like stress relief, sun exposure, and exercise, he continued to wear Ellen White's mantle of sexual suppression and strongly advocated limited meat consumption, all while extolling the benefits of fiber-rich plant foods for his patients, because he felt five bowel movements per day was the best way to rid the body of disease-causing bacteria. Kellogg's meat-phobia is also largely responsible for the myth that meat rots in the colon, which I'll discuss later.

Kellogg, known as an "incorrigible publicity hound," was driven by ego: Between 1875 and 1940, he recorded and sold his thoughts on topics of health through his own popular magazine, *Good Health,* through pamphlets, and through books marketed door to door. His "zealous efforts to proselytize the world at large," as the description of the John Harvey Kellogg Papers at the University of Michigan puts it, were conducted aggressively and continuously. And by *continuously,* I mean continuously: Kellogg wouldn't even go to the bathroom without a stenographer. Maybe because he spent the "bulk" of his fiber-filled time there. (Wink. Poop joke.)

In a modern world full of reality television and self-aggrandizing celebrity doctors, fitness trainers, and nutrition book writers (ha!), we can surely understand the concept of aggressive self-promotion. Kellogg managed to become world famous, even without the power of the Internet, through what the University of Michigan describes as his "vigorous efforts as a promoter and publicist." Kellogg was a successful propagandist who managed to spread his beliefs across the world, and while we remember his name thanks to his co-discovery of cornflakes (a product his brother was left to develop and market), and although this discovery grew from his vegetarian values, cereal is a very small part of his legacy.

What Kellogg truly left behind was the framework for modern-day vegetarianism. Though his last name isn't synonymous with that movement, he certainly played a powerful role in its development. He believed that humans should emulate the higher primates—gorillas and orangutans—by emphasizing a diet of grains, fruit, and nuts. He was among the early advocates of the development of "meat analogs" (or "fakin' bacon," as I like to call them), and he developed meat substitutes beginning with the peanut-based Protose in 1899, followed by the nut-based Nuttose and Nuttelene.

Today, the most widely known vegetarian protein source, which appears in everything from plant-based bacon bits to vegan sausage, is soy—which Kellogg predicted would become hugely important in America. Although Kellogg developed probiotic soy milk (I would argue that any supposed benefits attributed to the milk should have been attributed to the probiotics that came with it) and encouraged the incorporation of soybeans into the diet as a source of protein, the technology for mass-producing edible soy protein was not widely used until the late 1950s, when solvent extraction of soy oil was introduced. This industrial process allowed the protein-rich by-product of soy oil production to remain intact, enabling the isolated soy protein fibers to be texturized into a meat-like consistency.

It's interesting to note the inbreeding: The margarine industry, born of animal-product scarcity and saddled with trans fats, morphed into a crop oil industry with an anti-animal fat agenda; and the by-products from these industries provide the raw materials for the "fake meat" market and the factory-farming industry. Remember, the by-products of margarine production helped establish the feedlot industry, and most modern soy is used to produce animal feed for that same enterprise.

And all of us, in some way and at some point in our lives, have probably bought into that incestuous circle. Ew.

Unlike Kellogg's, our moral attitudes toward sex and masturbation today have little to do with our choice in foods (with a few naughty exceptions). Even so, our cultural enthusiasm for meatlessness has increased. Why? Part of the reason is that history is written by the winners—or at least by those who find a way, through ego or sheer enthusiasm, to foist their personal agendas and theories on the public.

I'm talking about Kellogg and antifat crusader Ancel Keys and the industries that were built up around them. You may have noticed that nearly everything with a label has a corn or soy by-product in it, and cornflakes are a mainstay of supermarket shelves, as are their by-product brethren, vegetable oils. These products are even considered by some to be healthy, although I would debate that wholeheartedly.

Let's quickly revisit the truth about cholesterol and foods rich in saturated fats from properly raised creatures: Not only are they not dangerous, they're actually extremely dense in nutrition. And while we probably don't need to further ridicule Kellogg's sex-drive-dampening dietary devotions (too easy—where's the fun?), we certainly can credit his work, along with that of Keys and researchers from the vegetable oil industry, in building the infrastructure for a modern meatless agenda that, at its core, has roots more deeply embedded in cardiovascular confusion and commerce than in true health. Massive industries arose around the shaky theories and questionable agendas of Keys and Kellogg, and their beliefs were inscribed in our cultural narrative. Other common arguments for a meatless diet are just fuel to a flame that should have died out long ago.

Though the evangelists of meatless nutrition have been loud throughout history, and their concerns about animal welfare are shared, albeit addressed differently, by compassionate omnivores dedicated to properly raised animal products (we'll talk about that), their proclamations can't mute the truth: We can't replace all animal products with plants and expect to get equal nutrition. Animals and plants are different outside our bodies, and they work differently within our bodies. One reason: protein. More specifically, amino acids.

The essentials on protein and amino acids

Proteins are made of varying combinations of amino acids, and amino acids make up every tissue and substance in our bodies, from hair to heart to hormones. We need the right combinations of amino acids interacting with fundamentally healthy cells in order to build tissues as nature intended. To misunderstand this is to misunderstand the roles that individual amino acids play in the growth, repair, and maintenance of healthy tissue. Amino acids matter.

There are eight essential amino acids for adults and nine for children. The body can make all other amino acids from these essential ones, but we must get the essential ones from the foods we consume.

Creature protein contains all the essential amino acids in proper proportion to one another—a characteristic of all flesh foods—and thus is known as *complete protein*. While all essential amino acids can also be found in the plant kingdom, they are not found in the same complete-protein proportions: Most plants provide inadequate amounts of certain amino acids in relation to others. For this reason, plant protein is known as *incomplete*. Although the meatless and the meat-full communities do not agree on the significance of this information, and many plant-based-diet devotees insist that the question of amino acid proportions doesn't matter, I aim to make clear that it does.

During the digestive process, our bodies free the amino acids within our food and create other substances from them. If something we eat doesn't contain the full suite of essential amino acids needed by the body, we have a very small window—one day by the estimation of the Centers for Disease Control and Prevention—to ingest the complementary ones to complete the amino acid equation. This is because the body doesn't house amino acids while they wait for their perfect counterparts to pass through. This ain't Match.com for amino acids.

The body doesn't store complete proteins for a rainy day, either. According to the Standing Committee on the Scientific Evaluation of Dietary Reference Intakes—or, as I like to call them, a bunch of awesome science nerds—"There is no evidence for a protein reserve that serves only as a store to meet future needs." Complete protein must be eaten daily to serve the body's ongoing needs, and those needs are many: tissue repair, the normal growth and development of a child, and the biochemical transactions that enable those tasks, from zinc and iron utilization to cholesterol-carrying to the building of proteins for oxygen transport. All depend on the amino acids found in protein. So, say the nerds, "The most important aspect of a protein from a nutritional point of view is its amino acid composition."

All this mumbo jumbo pertains most to those who rely primarily on plants for their amino acids with the false belief that protein is protein is protein, or the mistaken claim that the amino acid composition of protein doesn't matter. According to the nerds' analysis, "unless amino acids are present in the diet in the right balance . . . protein utilization will be affected." There are, in fact, consequences to relying exclusively on plants for protein, even if they aren't immediately recognizable. We may not be wasting away sans protein from animals or fish, but many of us are wasting perfectly good opportunities to feel better. We're also wasting a great opportunity to transform our food system by advocating for the humane treatment of animals by spending our food dollars on properly raised animal products—which I'll discuss later.

Let's look more deeply at the reasons so many people avoid creature protein. I've already noted the powerful roles that Kellogg and the vegetable oil industry played in shaping the conversation about animal products, but demolishing the puritanical and nutritionally unsound underpinnings of these industries doesn't extinguish the plant-based fire. The torch has been passed from religious crusaders and corporate insiders to well-meaning, compassionate, health-conscious individuals who have assembled a big-hearted goodie bag of objections to counter any inclination toward meat-eating.

What objections are these? In addition to the most common animal-eating admonition—that it's unhealthy—are contentions that meat consumption is environmentally unsound and, of course, that it's just plain mean to eat another sentient creature. Other objections abound, and they tend to come up in whack-a-mole succession. We're going to knock them all out. Clubs at the ready.

Myth:
Animal protein causes cancer

Having tackled the question of animal fats and the cardiovascular realm in chapter 1, it's now time to address the protein problem: the idea that animal protein is toxic to our bodies. For those entrenched in the old school (of hard arteries) way of thinking, it's an easy transition to make—if animal fat is bad for the body, animal protein should be, too.

And that's exactly what T. Colin Campbell claims in his book *The China Study*. Any omnivore who has discussed dietary habits with a veggivore will recognize the title, which is generally sandwiched breathlessly between "have you read" and "animal protein causes cancer."

The biggest problem with *The China Study* isn't that Campbell's writings have been called into question by scientists and keen-eyed laypeople alike for possible issues and omissions in his summarization of the data. (That's right—data was omitted, whether purposely or not.)

The biggest problem with *The China Study* isn't even that it's not a study. I repeat, it's not a study. It's simply a book title. The author of *The China Study*, T. Colin Campbell, was among several scientists involved with the China-Cornell-Oxford project, which, to its credit, actually was a study—an observational study on the diet and health of the people of sixty-five counties in rural China, with data gathered between 1983 and 1990, bound into an 894-page volume published in 1990 titled *Diet, Life-Style, and Mortality in China: A Study of the Characteristics of 65 Chinese Counties*. In 2004, quite a few years later, *The China Study* was published. It devotes just a fraction of its pages to the study to which its name alludes; the rest of it focuses on other experiments Campbell conducted on laboratory rats over the course of several decades.

The biggest problem with *The China Study* is that it gives the reader nothing more than a poorly backed sound bite that turns out to be a completely mangled take on the truth. A meaner way to say this is: It makes Tofurkeys out of its toadies.

There is no proof in any of Campbell's research that animal protein causes cancer. In fact, Campbell's own research, both his work in China and his later experiments with rats—especially the parts he omitted from his own book on the topic—make this quite clear.

Why isn't this common knowledge? Because it's not easy, it's not what the author wanted to tell us, and it's not what we wanted to hear.

But the facts can't be ignored. In separate, comprehensive audits, nutrition experts Loren Cordain, Chris Masterjohn, Anthony Colpo, and Denise Minger looked at the source material for *The China Study,* the China-Cornell-Oxford Project itself, and Campbell's data from experiments on rats, and they all found some very unfortunate details of scientific ball-dropping.

As Denise Minger reported in her comprehensive critique of *The China Study,* the observational data from the China-Cornell-Oxford project published in *Diet, Life-Style, and Mortality in China: A Study of the Characteristics of 65 Chinese Counties* actually found a closer association not between animal protein and cancer but between *plant* protein and cancer. And heart disease. And stroke. It also showed a much stronger association between wheat and heart disease mortality.

These associations were, unfortunately, not discussed in *The China Study.*

To be fair, observational data can be affected by any number of complications. Environmental factors from smog to soil health, lifestyle factors from smoking to exercise, and other nutritional factors, from vitamins to trace mineral intake, can all interfere with our ability to paint a clear picture of what might—or might not—cause a particular health problem. The takeaway here, though, is that Campbell's conclusions, like Keys's, were drawn against undeniably, obviously, clearly contradictory evidence. And that's not cool.

Remember, there are two parts to *The China Study:* the small portion devoted to the China-Cornell-Oxford project and the part built upon Campbell's experiments on laboratory rats. Knowing that animal protein does not correlate most strongly with cancer in the China-Cornell-Oxford project data, it's not particularly shocking that the lab rat results don't stand up to scrutiny, either. Whether we look at the human data (the observations of rural Chinese people) or the lab-tested data (the controlled experiments on rats), the science doesn't support a causal relationship between animal protein and cancer.

What really happened in the lab (or, I smell a rat)

Between approximately 1972 and 1994, Campbell tested what he believed to be a connection between animal protein and cancer with a fairly uniform approach over the course of multiple studies. Rats were poisoned with a fungus-derived toxin that must be processed through the liver. At different points before, during, and after their poisoning, these rats were fed solutions containing casein, an incomplete animal-based protein found in milk. Some rats received more casein in their feeding solution, and some received less. Some of the poisoned rats that were given the solution with more casein developed liver cancer and cancerlike markers. If we're to believe Campbell, since casein is an animal-derived protein, this is evidence that animal protein promotes cancer. Campbell offers this interpretation of his studies, and the study they were based upon, in *The China Study*.

Yet there are several things that didn't make it into the book.

First, according to Masterjohn, the poisoned rats that had less casein in their feeding solution didn't skip away, singing and holding hands. What Campbell failed to state in his book—although the evidence was present in his own research—is that these rats experienced tissue damage and liver cell death, among other problems. They may not have developed liver cancer, but they still suffered major health problems. Like cell death. Their cells were dying.

Masterjohn also uncovered that the casein in Campbell's experiments was supplemented with an additional amino acid, making it not just casein anymore. Remember, proteins are built from combinations of amino acids. Adding an

amino acid to an existing protein creates an entirely different protein. If your lab experiment aims to prove something
about casein, you should probably use—I dunno—casein.

While these teensy-weensy little facts were included in
Campbell's original body of research, somehow they didn't
make it into *The China Study*.

Most important, it wasn't even the casein solutions, demonized for their animal origins, that were uniquely associated with problems. Campbell achieved equivalent results
when he used wheat protein supplemented with an additional amino acid. Whether the protein was from animals or
plants, the results were similar when an additional amino
acid was added.

What were these additional amino acids, and what enabled them to wreak their havoc on these poor, innocent rats?

These extra amino acids were added to make the incomplete proteins in each experiment—casein protein and
wheat protein—complete. Think back to our discussion of
what makes a protein complete: It's the presence of all essential amino acids. In Campbell's studies, the addition of
amino acids to both the incomplete animal-derived protein
(casein) and the incomplete plant-derived protein (wheat gluten) brought each of those proteins to a complete state—all
essential amino acids were now present. Whether the complete protein was of plant or animal origin didn't matter. All
essential amino acids were present and accounted for, and
although it isn't mentioned in *The China Study*, all the rats
experienced some type of health problem, whether they were
fed more or less complete protein.

Does this mean that all my yammering about the importance of complete proteins is balderdash? That complete
proteins—whether we get them from animals or plants and
in any amount, small or large—cause health problems, and
we should actually avoid them entirely?

No! Remember, Campbell's rats were not only sick when
they were fed complete protein; they were also sick on

incomplete protein. They were sick on more of it and they were sick on less of it. They were sick on both animal- and plant-derived protein, too. Why? Because before they were fed any of it, they were poisoned!

Because protein provides the raw materials for structure and growth, more protein stimulated the growth of the rats' poisoned tissues, leading to tumors and cancer. Less protein—which could also be termed *protein deficiency*—caused the opposite effect: The rats' cells died. Why? Because they didn't have enough protein to maintain their own structure.

The problem wasn't the complete proteins. Feeding rats more complete protein, in fact, did exactly what it was supposed to do: provide the raw materials for growth. Feeding cancer makes it grow, just like watering a weed makes the weed thrive. Does that mean water causes weeds? No. (But it may mean you suck at gardening. Okay, it may mean I suck at gardening.)

If you keep your garden free of weeds, they won't overwhelm what you're actually trying to grow. Campbell's own experiments indicated that rats fed a higher-protein solution *before* being poisoned—as in rats who were given the raw materials for fighting toxic exposures—were actually protected against cancer.

We want healthy cells to grow, which implies the need for—duh—healthy cells. Healthy cells are free of the influence of, say, fungus-derived toxins like those used to poison the rats in Campbell's experiments. We can achieve this not by eschewing protein but by not poisoning ourselves with fungus-derived toxins and then encouraging manipulated cells to thrive. Seems intuitive enough.

Maybe that's the real sound bite from *The China Study:* Don't get poisoned in the first place!

This is not an indictment of the author of *The China Study* or those who follow its advice, although it likely sounds that way. Campbell's scientific achievements are vast and admirable, but that doesn't change the facts: There's more to the story—in places, there's an entirely different story—than the one we've been told, and the more context we have, the easier this is to understand. Campbell—who, like me, advocates eating real, unprocessed foods, albeit not those from animals—simply didn't prove that animal protein is inherently dangerous.

There is another side of that coin, however, and it needs to be said: Though animal protein is not harmful, not all animal *products* are created equal. Much more comes along with the protein we eat than simply amino acids, and animals raised in unnatural, abusive factory farms, also known as feedlots or Concentrated Animal Feeding Operations (CAFOs), are as unhealthy as the environment in which they live and the foods—industrial crops—they're force-fed. We are what we eat—so we want to eat healthy, properly raised animals. I'll get to that, too.

But first, let's address another animal-protein myth that is no more true for having been repeated thousands of times: the idea that protein is, in various ways, hard on the body—the kidneys, the liver, and the bones. It's just not true.

Myth: Animal protein is bad for the kidneys, liver, and bones

These theories, which have exceedingly poor evidence to support them and far more evidence to discredit them, are repeated in books and blogs, echoed by medical professionals and laypeople alike, and treated as foregone conclusions. They likely grew legs (or stems, depending on your inclination) not for their strong body of proof—it doesn't exist—but because of a fundamental misunderstanding of the way our bodies digest and handle the protein we eat. That misunderstanding has been compounded by the social and institutional acceptance of the supposed dangers of meat-eating. Hitching a ride with that dogma, these ideas about how protein hurts the liver, kidneys, and bones wobbled awkwardly under the falling limbo stick of the dietary myths of the last half-century. (Truly, is there any other way to do the limbo?)

Here's how protein is used in the body, which gives some hints as to why the protein-kidney-liver myths have had some staying power: Protein, whether from animals or plants, is our only dietary source of nitrogen, which is used to build the raw materials for everything from blood to hair to DNA. To extract and use that nitrogen, the body employs a process that generates a waste product called ammonia. The liver must convert ammonia to urea, which is then excreted by the kidneys through urine. If you believe the hype, this is too demanding a process for our bodies to handle.

But just because protein makes demands on the liver and kidneys, does this mean that protein is hard on them? Absolutely not, but I suppose being entrenched in the standard dogma about the connection between animal products, heart disease, and cancer might have made us more amenable to the myth. The truth, however, is that processing the vital nitrogen in dietary protein is the job of the liver and kidneys—a very important one—and healthy livers and kidneys gotta earn their keep somehow. We'd never believe that using our brains or muscles less could make them better able to do their jobs, but we've somehow decided that the liver and kidneys should be treated like the boss's kid, tasked with as little as possible and allowed to sit in the corner office playing Minesweeper all day.

There's no evidence to support putting these organs on a reduced schedule. A study comparing long-term vegetarians who had low relative protein intake with a group of meat-eaters showed absolutely no difference in kidney function between the two groups. A separate study by Megan A. Kniskern and Carol S. Johnston did emphasize potential problems with a vegetarian diet, though, stating that "long-term adherence to [vegetarian] diets may be associated with nutrient inadequacies, particularly vitamins B_{12} and D, calcium, iron, zinc, and protein." The protein deficiency was attributed to the "decreased protein bioavailability" of plants—yet another argument for getting protein from healthy creatures raised in their natural environments on their natural diets.

A published analysis of the body of scientific literature on protein intake and liver, kidney, and bone health indicates that "there is no scientific evidence whatsoever that high-protein intake has adverse effects on liver function." With regard to kidney function, the analysis states, "There are no data in the scientific literature demonstrating that healthy kidneys are damaged by the increased demands of protein consumed in quantities 2–3 times above the Recommended Dietary Allowance (RDA)."

The key phrase in that sentence is *healthy kidneys.* While protein can't be held responsible for *causing* kidney problems, if a kidney issue already exists, it makes sense that the kidneys would be less able to do the job of excreting urea. A person with a broken leg can't be expected to run the hundred-yard dash, and a diabetic can't be expected to tolerate carbohydrates the same way a person with a normal pancreas could.

And protein can't be blamed for the development of liver or kidney problems, either. Evidence indicates that chronically high blood sugar and hypertension are actually correlated with kidney disease. (They're also correlated with diabetes, erectile dysfunction, stroke, depression, and obesity, but let's not get greedy.) Dietary protein intake, however, has been tied to reduced blood pressure and better blood-sugar management—meaning that protein could actually protect the kidneys from problems associated with high blood sugar.

Animal products, especially nutrient-dense animal fat, may even be necessary for healthy kidney function. Masterjohn suggests that a deficiency in the animal-derived form of vitamin K_2 is a major cause of kidney stones, since vitamin K_2 helps tell the body where to lay down calcium. (I'll discuss K_2 further in chapter 4.) Vitamin K_2 is found in fats from grass-fed ruminants, especially their milk fat. Have I encouraged you to eat butter yet?

Speaking of calcium, here's where things really get fun. The myth that animal protein is hard on the bones, which are the source of our vital calcium reserves, grew from the fact that protein from animals contains acidic compounds, like sulfur, and the myth that the body must pull calcium from the bones to buffer the acidic effects of animal protein on the body. (Fun fact: Most whole grains and legumes are also acidic, so an animal-protein-free diet based around the full complement of amino acids could be equally "acidic.")

The idea that acid is bad and alkaline is good is simple—too simple, unfortunately, to accord with the truth about how our bodies work. Animal proteins are, indeed, rich in sulfur-containing amino acids, and sulfur is incredibly important for our health—it plays a role in our bodies' critical antioxidants as well as vitamin D metabolism and hair and skin health. Fruits and vegetables, by contrast, are rich in compounds of alkaline pH. These compounds are also healthful.

When it comes to bone health and all the acid-alkaline chatter floating through the nutrisphere, we've held on to major misconceptions, even though Robert P. Heaney, "the author of the most cited paper favoring the . . . hypothesis that high-protein intake promotes osteoporosis, no longer believes that protein is harmful to bone." Heaney himself has concluded that the evidence points to the entirely opposite conclusion—that animal protein supports bone health. He has further indicated that the zeal for vegan and vegetarian diets and "eagerness to exploit any evidence that suggests harmful effects of animal products" may have been responsible for this enthusiastic misrepresentation of scientific evidence.

A 2011 analysis in *Current Opinion in Lipidology* states that "epidemiological, isotopic and meta-analysis studies" (meaning "pretty much all the science ever") indicate that dietary protein works with the calcium in the body, not against it. The science shows that dietary protein actually helps improve calcium retention and bone health—and the analysis goes on to caution that restricting dietary protein based on bone health concerns could even be dangerous.

So what's the deal with acidic foods, then, and how do our bodies process them? Here's where we get to ooh and aah over the amazing built-in mechanisms our bodies have for digesting and using the healthy foods we're meant to eat. In the conversion of critical nitrogen to ammonia to urea, the body creates bicarbonate, which neutralizes acid all by itself. Hooray—the acidic foods we eat actually buffer themselves.

Just as it is the job of the muscles to move, lift, and pull, and just as it is the job of the stomach to aid in the digestion of food, it is the job of the kidneys to process components in protein, the job of the liver to manage substances circulating in the body, and the job of the bones to maintain their strength. Asking our tissues to do their jobs—jobs that allow us to build other tissues, deploy substances essential for health, and maintain homeostasis—does not burden them. It fulfills their biological purpose.

Myth: We can get all the protein we need from plants

Protein is more complex than we imagine it to be. While, strictly speaking, an egg or a tin of sardines could have the same quantity of protein as a serving of cereal or a bowl of beans, the quality of that protein is vastly different.

Proteins from different sources, as we've discussed, have different amino acids. More important, they have different amounts of essential amino acids, the ones our bodies need to get from food. Protein from plants tends to be lacking in one or more essential amino acids, making it "incomplete." Protein sources also provide other nutrients and compounds, of course, and in the case of popular plant-based sources of protein, these include antinutrients—substances that prevent the body from absorbing nutrients effectively. Antinutrients make many plant-based protein sources less digestible, less nutrient-dense, and more problematic than their creature counterparts.

When we rely solely on plants for our protein, amino acid imbalance can also become a problem, since we're not getting the complete proteins that we get from animals. For example, wheat is low in tryptophan, which is abundant in creature foods and provides the necessary ingredients for serotonin, a neurotransmitter that helps regulate mood and sleep. Corn is low in tryptophan and lysine, a component in collagen that is also abundant in properly raised creature foods.

Tyrosine, which is created from phenylalanine, an essential amino acid found in animal protein, provides the building blocks for thyroid hormones and dopamine. Taurine, a derivative compound of the amino acid cysteine (found in—you guessed it—animal foods), is a building block for bile, which allows us to digest nutritious, delicious fat—and the nutrients that come with it.

Despite all this, none of the problems of total reliance on plant protein are likely to cause immediate, glaring issues for a plants-only eater. Heads won't explode and hair won't fall out (at least not right away). Further, even if deficiencies become extreme and severe symptoms manifest, there are few issues connected to amino acid deficiencies that we can't treat medically without ever thinking about what caused the issue in the first place. If we have depression due to serotonin deficiency, we take antidepressants. If we have anxiety or connective tissue breakdown due to lysine deficiency, we take antianxiety pills or wear Spanx (been there, done that).

Point is, our lives are flooded with foods, supplements, and consumables (including prescriptions) of all kinds, available any time we want them, and many of them compensate for the shortcomings of the others. Without this level of consumerism, absent a change in our food paradigm (which I advocate), our lives might be very different. Here's an example of how critical the proper balance of amino acids is in a more controlled environment: Pet foods are crafted to extreme specifications to ensure that Fido gets the right profile of amino acids (whether through a combination of low-grade plant protein or actual meat) because animals don't have the same free-consuming lives as we do. They can't compensate for amino acid imbalance as we can with a pill or a secret steak.

There are, admittedly, whole-plant exceptions to the complete protein conundrum. One of them is soy, which is technically considered complete even though, next to animal protein, it's comparatively low in the sulfur-containing essential amino acid methionine, which is critical in all aspects of cell metabolism. (And sulfur itself is emerging as an incredibly critical nutrient for human health.) But soy—like other plants, including those high in protein—is equipped with defense mechanisms against those who would eat it. In soy, these mechanisms are hormone-manipulating substances, such as goitrogens and phytoestrogens, and protease inhibitors, which inhibit the digestion of the amino acid cysteine and thereby prevent the body from using it to build taurine, which is also emerging as a critical nutrient for human health. (Plants'll getcha. They might not be able to run, kick, or bite, but they'll getcha.)

This says nothing about the fact that soy is, for the most part, genetically modified. But it's all connected, undeniably, intricately, inescapably, and in ways that are still being revealed.

Now, before I move on, I'll devote exactly as much time as deserved to the highly trafficked plant protein aisles at your local high-end grocer. With regards to hemp, chia, rice, spirulina, quinoa, lentils, peas, chlorella, beans, protein powders, and, as the King of Siam would say, et cetera, et cetera, et cetera: Have the heck at 'em. They are not inherently harmful foods. Some of them are even complete proteins. Some of them, however, are just by-products of industries that are lucky enough to have the powers of a marketing department behind them. Much of the market for them is driven by an unfounded fear of hearty, healthy animal products, and though a few are nutritious, they are not more nutritious than those staple creature foods that carry such a broad spectrum of the nutrients we need. They serve as tired distractions from the real questions: Is our current dietary dogma founded on a pack of lies? And are creature foods nutritious or pernicious?

I'm not harping on this just 'cause I want to justify my unabashed affinity for surf 'n' turf. In all honesty, I've always liked rice and beans darn near as much. But it's a simple fact of life that when it comes to amino acids, creature protein contains all of what's needed, and plant protein, with a few rare exceptions, does not. Traditional cultures around the world have understood this for thousands of years, valuing animal foods above all other protein sources and, when animal foods are scarce, constructing a diet that mimics their amino acid composition.

Many will recognize this concept—now known as *protein combining*—without realizing that it's not just a developed-world idea. It's a concept that, in resource-bound cultures, was born of ancestral wisdom in times of scarcity. There's a reason that certain cultures combined incomplete proteins from plants like rice, corn, or beans in traditional dishes. It's because creature protein wasn't always available, and rice, for example, happens to contain the amino acids lacking in beans (and vice versa).

It's unlikely that we'd recognize any immediate symptoms of amino acid imbalance after eating, for example, beans without rice. We're an instant-gratification society, and if something doesn't immediately decimate us like a wooden stake in a vampire's cold, dead heart, we generally assume we're okay. If we're tired, run-down, or listless, or we poop out at parties, we don't attribute that to amino acid imbalance or nutrient deficiency. It's just how we happen to feel that day. So we take a shot of 5-Hour Energy—which is full of complementary amino acids and B vitamins, just like you'd find in a steak—perk right up, and move on, none the wiser.

In truth, protein combining may not even matter in today's Western world, which is flooded with food, supplements, and deficiency-masking pharmaceuticals of every kind. Even the modern developed-world articulator of the protein-combining philosophy, Frances Moore Lappé (author of *Diet for a Small Planet*), reconsidered and eventually recanted her position that combining is important to strategizing modern life sans meat. Yet traditional cultures still did it, and even if we choose to ignore the issue of individual amino acids and where we get them, we can certainly learn something from our ancestors, who never went without creature foods intentionally or entirely.

What exactly can we learn from them? Perhaps that the benefits of creature foods are greater than the sum of their amino acids.

Here's the question that inevitably arises from that statement: If that's true, then why are vegetarians so much healthier than meat-eaters?

They're not.

Salad or steak?
Vegetarianism and your health

Though shocking headlines linking meat-eating to chronic disease have received attention of late, upon closer investigation, we find that there is more to the story. It turns out that, according to a study published in *Circulation,* processed meat—the kind rich in synthetic nitrates and preservatives—"but not red meats, is associated with higher incidence of [coronary heart disease] and diabetes mellitus."

This brings up an issue of scientific rigor that was discussed in the introduction. Lumping together people with one thing in common—say, eating meat—in an effort to draw a conclusion about the group's overall health status may still mean haphazardly grouping together people with vastly different dietary habits. For example, a group designated as "meat-eaters" could be composed of both those who chow down on factory-farmed meats laden with artificial preservatives and those who choose their properly raised meats carefully, avoiding synthetic preservatives altogether. Likewise, a group designated as "vegetarian" could be composed of people who eat whole, unrefined foods and organically grown fruits and vegetables as well as those vegetarians who huff processed soy meat substitutes within flour- and trans fat–filled buns. To make reasonable comparisons between vegetarians and meat-eaters requires grouping test subjects based on—well, common sense. This means taking into account similarities in lifestyle, not just using a dietary designation that could have multiple manifestations.

Which is what one study published in the *International Journal of Behavioral Nutrition and Physical Activity* did. "Taken as a whole," it concluded, "studies have shown that vegetarians are in good physical health compared with national averages and as healthy as nonvegetarians *with a comparable background and lifestyle*" (emphasis mine). The health-conscious, whether vegetarian or not, were found to be equally healthy—physically, at least.

The mental health of vegetarians was not observed to be as robust. The same study stated that "people suffering from a mental disorder ate less meat than people without a mental disorder." One explanation for this is that having a mental disorder may increase the likelihood of eliminating meat from one's diet. A more likely explanation: Deficiencies in nutrients found in animal products that are critical for mental health—nutrients like cholesterol, vitamin B_{12}, the amino acid methionine, and many others—may increase the likelihood of developing mental health problems.

Certain nutrients found in animal products work synergistically to regulate mood- and mental health–related physiology. The process of methylation, which regulates dopamine—a compound that is crucial for healthy brain function—is dependent on methionine, glycine, vitamin B_{12}, and folate, which are all found in creature foods. A marker of glycine deficiency is the urinary excretion of oxoproline, and vegetarians have been found to have twice as much oxoproline in their urine as omnivores.

This inspires the question: What other nutrients might be missing from a meatless diet?

The benefits of animal products
(or, nose-to-tail never fails)

Animal protein does not occur alone in nature. While a steak contains complete protein, it also contains fat, vitamin A, B vitamins, iron, zinc, and cholesterol. It is attached to bones and connective tissue, which are reservoirs of minerals, gelatin, and glycine. Organ meats are incredibly rich sources of B vitamins and trace minerals.

Of course, different creature proteins boast different nutrient densities. Chicken breast is one of the most nutrient-poor sources of complete protein around, not to mention that well-endowed chickens are almost always products of factory farms. (And our love affair with clucker boobage is just an offshoot of our fear of fat anyway.) The most nutrient-rich proteins are from properly raised or wild ruminant red meat, which is dense in zinc, iron, vitamin A, conjugated linoleic acid, and cholesterol. The most nutrient-filled seafood isn't farm-raised tilapia or overfished tuna but wild-caught salmon and oily, low-food-chain swimmers like sardines, which are rich in vitamin D, calcium, and taurine, and oysters, which are rich in zinc and cholesterol.

We'll talk more about vitamins A, D, and K and important minerals in chapter 4, but for now let's turn our attention to the most compelling argument for creature foods: vitamin B_{12}.

While it's easy (if shortsighted) to quash nutrition-related objections to vegetarianism when a nutrient is found in both plants and animals, as certain minerals and B vitamins are, dismissing the issue requires—and I say this with love—total commitment to dietary delusion when it comes to B_{12}.

B_{12} is found only in animal products, yet even lacto-ovo vegetarians (those who eat milk and eggs) may miss out on it. Surprised? Sometimes what matters most isn't whether a nutrient is found within a food but whether the body can actually absorb it and use it properly. According to a report in the *Journal of Experimental Biology and Medicine,* the bioavailability of vitamin B_{12} from eggs is less than 9 percent—meaning that of all the B_{12} found in eggs, the body absorbs only 9 percent. Compare that to the bioavailability of B_{12} found in red meat, which is as high as 77 percent. That's not to say eggs aren't incredibly nutritious—they are, the yolks in particular—but B_{12} isn't their banner nutrient. And when it comes to the "lacto" part of lacto-ovo vegetarianism, there's baggage as well: Due to high-temperature pasteurization, the structurally damaging homogenization process, and the improper care and feeding of most commercial dairy cows, most *lacto* is severely *lacking* in nutrients.

The lack of B_{12} in plants is a glaring issue that many devoted plants-only eaters are well prepared to refute with oft-repeated myths that make any concern seem hackneyed. To have an eye-roll response to a serious biological reality is—to quote *The Gods Must Be Crazy*—a very interesting psychological phenomenon. (An apt phrase, since B_{12} is as vital to mental health as it is to physical health.)

The most common claims about B_{12} on a completely creature-free diet are, first, that we can obtain it from certain plants, and second, that we don't need much of it anyway.

Vitamin B_{12} is derived from bacteria. It's even made by the bacteria in our own colons, although that stuff isn't reabsorbed directly back into our bodies (since B_{12} is absorbed earlier in the digestive tract). A small group of cultural vegans in Iran were found to maintain B_{12} sufficiency by growing plants in human feces—dubbed *night soil*—and not fully washing away this special fertilizer before eating. Something to think about, I guess.

B_{12} is absolutely not derived from plants. "There is no active vitamin B-12 in anything that grows out of the ground," says physician and nutrition expert Victor Herbert in the *American Journal of Clinical Nutrition.* "Storage vitamin B-12 is found only in animal products where it is ubiquitous and where it is ultimately derived from bacteria."

The body can store and recycle B_{12}, which is indeed good news should we ever find ourselves locked in a hydroponic greenhouse. In extreme circumstances, it makes sense to have this adaptation—B_{12} is so necessary that our bodies evolved the capacity to store it for survival in times of scarcity. However, there's a downside: Our ability to store B_{12} means that the symptoms of long-term inadequate intake can take years to manifest, and by the time they do, it's too late. Surviving is very different from thriving, and risking B_{12} deficiency means risking loss of the myelin sheath that insulates our nerves, nerve degeneration, mental disturbance, pernicious anemia, muscle stiffness and spasms, impotence, and loss of sensation in the extremities. Once these symptoms manifest, it's nearly impossible to fully recover.

Even Gabriel Cousens, a physician and longtime "live food" vegan advocate, cautions vegans about the extreme dangers of B_{12} deficiency on a vegan diet and advocates taking B_{12} supplements. And according to Herbert, studies indicate that *all* strict vegans eventually develop "vitamin B-12 deficiency disease with anemia and pancytopenia, low white counts, low red counts, low platelet counts, and slowed DNA synthesis . . . which is corrected by vitamin B-12."

Although several edible algae, including chlorella, are known to carry active vitamin B_{12}, they also may contain inactive B_{12} analogues that compete with active B_{12} for assimilation. Other algae that contain B_{12}, including spirulina, contain inactive analogues of the vitamin.

Remember those pesky plant goitrogens, which can interfere with thyroid function? This would likely prove less problematic for an omnivore than for a vegetarian, since B_{12} is used to detoxify goitrogens from the body.

When we choose to depart fully from ways of eating so firmly grounded in historical tradition and nutritional biochemistry, we had damn well better understand the potential consequences of trading flesh for forage. Neither health misinformation nor emotionally driven meatlessness can make us immune to the biological intricacies involved in processes like methylation, dopamine regulation, homocysteine conversion, and nervous system function, all of which require B_{12} to work properly. Just because you're lookin' the other way doesn't mean the car won't hit ya.

Living entirely on plant foods is a choice made possible only by the constant supply line of the modern supermarket. Vitamin B_{12} supplements, not to mention year-round produce and other plant foods that require good weather and, often, heavy pesticides to ensure their survival and worldwide shipping routes to ensure their supply, are modern conveniences.

Our ancestors understood how vital creature foods were to their health, so much so that they considered them sacred. (This thoughtful approach is, admittedly, missing in the social current surrounding meat-eating today.) Whether they consume insects, organ meat, sea creatures, or more conventional cuts of meat, cultures across the globe and throughout history have made use of creature nutrition in some way, shape, or form.

So how much meat do I gotta eat?

You may notice that I don't editorialize about how much creature protein we need. Why? Because it depends. What are you building? Are you a growing kid, a pregnant woman, a bodybuilder, or a couch potato? Truth is, I don't care how much you eat. I care about quality and nutrient density. The rest, I believe, generally works itself out.

And, as I'm not here to advocate some dogmatic high-protein-or-die diet, let me say this: Depending on your stage of life and physical condition, you may need less total protein relative to others. The typical Atkins dieter, for example, eats more total protein than our minimum biological requirement for reasons of appetite control, not amino acid sufficiency.

Yet if we look at our protein status like a checking account, it's much better to aim for more generous deposits—not Trump-esque chunks of change, but enough to feel comfortable—so that we can make withdrawals and call upon the requisite amino acids and nutrients as needed. This is because we absolutely cannot predict our protein, nutrient, or amino acid needs moment by moment, and an argument over the average person's protein need is just that—an argument over an average, which doesn't account for the tasks assigned to individual amino acids in the first place. Simply squeaking by with the bare minimum to prevent amino acid deficiency does nothing to ensure robust health.

Making sure we have enough protein in the bank doesn't mean eating a full cow at every meal, but it does mean not falling for low-protein proselytizing. Protein and the nutrients that should come packaged with it are too important to skimp on for the sake of guilt or oversimplified, shortsighted information—like the flat-out lie that animal protein turns us into disease-ridden fleshophiles; the mistaken idea that all protein is the same, whatever the source; or the false claim that, because of a perceived similarity to our distant primate relatives, we can't digest creature foods properly in the first place.

Myth: We need to eat like primates (or, don't monkey around with ape food)

·····································

There is a persistent myth—one Kellogg helped origi-nate—that we're best equipped to eat the same foods as our closest nonhuman relatives. Because this myth is often in-tertwined with the argument that raw foodism is the ideal diet—presumably because it's closest to an ape's diet, but more likely because it also tends to cause weight loss, the holy grail of diet culture—I'll tackle these myths together.

Here's the deal, and it's pretty simple: Cooking causes structural changes to food that enable us *Homo sapiens,* with our big cerebral cortex and ability to reason, to extract more energy and more nutrition from it. Raw foodists are gener-ally thin because uncooked food provides lower nutrient bio-availability—fewer calories—than the same food cooked, and it's incredibly difficult to eat enough raw plant food to get suf-ficient calories to fuel the body. This certainly causes weight loss, but does it provide overall, long-term health gains? Not so much.

We often confuse "thin" with "healthy" and "healthy diet" with "intervention diet," but losing weight on any given diet doesn't make that diet—or the person losing weight—health-ier in the long term. Case in point: Modern meat-free raw foodists of low body weight, both male and female, have been observed to have poor or nonexistent reproductive func-tion—men become impotent and women cease menstruat-ing. This is *the* health red flag, as the ability to reproduce is one of the clearest markers of biological fitness. Given that it's nearly impossible to consume adequate calories and, by extension, adequate nutrients from raw plant food, the ex-treme consequences that can result from low body weight and lower nutrient reserves are unavoidable long-term risks of this type of diet. Trading a few extra vanity pounds for infertility seems like a bad deal to me. A raw-food diet may help us be skinny (and if I were a raw foodist, I probably *would* be a "skinny bitch," not to mention a hungry one), but it is not a guarantee of great health.

Without the modern supermarket or, for the more self-sufficient raw foodist, the modern gardening supply store and several acres on which to cultivate plant foods, the ability to ensure a steady stream of less-extractable calories (a waste of potential nutrition, if you ask me) is not so simple. Two thousand calories of even the most energy-dense raw food, such as a banana, still has fewer nutrients than an equal amount of organ meat or fat-rich creature food cooked using the other human innovation that sets us apart from apes: fire.

Harvard anthropologist Richard Wrangham has said that he has "not been able to find any reports of people living long term on raw wild food." It is cooking, Wrangham contends, that enabled us to increase our brain capacity at the expense of a plant-exclusive gut. When we began cooking, we diverted energy toward brain development and away from the laborious and energy-intensive process of metabolizing raw plant matter. And our digestive systems evolved accordingly.

Cooking marks our departure from our primate ancestors. It let us make more out of less. While raw food–eating primates spent most of their days seeking, chewing, and digesting food, humans were able to spend time honing skills, transitioning from hunting and gathering to pastoralism and farming, and cultivating the other things that make us unique, such as art, architecture, and religion. (By the way, I use the term *cooking* loosely, as my own skills haven't evolved much from the basic application of fire. I burn things.)

Because cooking food makes calories more bioavailable, thousands of years of making use of fire has caused our digestive systems to evolve differently from those of primates. Our mouths and jaws are smaller and less powerful, our stomachs are smaller, and our digestive systems are, Wrangham says, "less than 60 percent of the mass that would be expected for a primate of our body weight." We've evolved over thousands of years to digest cooked food, whether animal or plant.

As a result, our shorter human colon makes us unable to digest large volumes of fibrous plant matter as apes can. This is likely due to a gradual evolutionary progression away from the metabolic cost of digesting raw plant matter. Digesting lots of raw plants takes a ton of energy, so cooking gave us an evolutionary advantage that ultimately changed the human colon to be quite different from that of apes. "Thanks to cooking," says Wrangham, "very high-fiber food of a type eaten by great apes is no longer a useful part of our diet."

We move, live, and function quite differently from apes, and our plant-digesting capacity—or lack thereof—reflects that evolutionary separation. The false argument that our digestive system is similar to that of primates—or any large creature that is not human—seems to persist only as a defense of a meatless diet rich in raw plants.

Katharine Milton, a professor of anthropology at the University of California–Berkeley, draws further distinctions between human and primate guts, stating that the human small intestine has evolved to digest a diet of nutritionally concentrated creature foods rather than plants, while the ape colon has evolved to digest copious plant matter that can't be digested in the small intestine. Apes, unlike humans, have a "voluminous hindgut" that functions to ferment—as in, further digest—large volumes of plant matter.

The term *fermentation* brings me to an essential item of bull-you-know-what that makes me want to go ape-you-know-what every time I hear it: the argument that flesh foods rot in the human colon. We absolutely can and do digest meat effectively, and the idea that meat "rots" in the colon is easily quashed by a quick lesson in human physiology—one that Kellogg, who disseminated this myth, clearly wasn't too concerned about.

Here's the short lesson: The digestive tract isn't a pipe that runs directly from top to tail, delivering chewed-up food to the hind parts to rot until our morning trip to the can. It's actually designed, by some miracle, to digest food. And digest it, it does.

Here's the long lesson: Every step in the digestive process is designed to do an important job. The saliva in our mouths and the act of chewing break down food physically. The incredibly acidic pH of the stomach and its churning action are designed to continue breaking down foods, especially proteins, which enables us to use the amino acids they contain. From there, enzymes further break down proteins and carbohydrates, while other enzymes and bile break down fats. All the while, hormones like gastrin, insulin, and glucagon tell the body what to do with all the nutrients we take in. These nutrients are absorbed in the small intestine through the action of the villi, tiny hairlike protrusions that pull nutrients into circulation.

Every digestive step utilizes a specific substance or group of substances to break down the foods we eat. Once food reaches the colon, we're looking at one substance in particular or, more accurately, one teeming microbiome filled with billions of bacteria, sometimes known as *probiotics,* whose primary function is to break down insoluble fiber, any intact starches, and cellulose from the plants we eat.

Meat is actually disassembled and assimilated long before it reaches the end of the digestive road. It does not rot in the colon. But plants sure do. In fact, the bacteria in the colon is our only hope for the full digestion of those plants, because without this hot colonic rot action, the cellulose we eat wouldn't be digested at all. (Tell me again that meat is harder to digest than plants. I dare ya.) And sometimes, despite the rigorous digestive process, plant foods still aren't completely digested. I've never seen a steak make its way intact from top to tail, but anyone who's eaten a batch of kale or corn will recognize its second commode-coming.

No animal has the ability to digest the plant fiber cellulose solely through its own—ahem—secretions, but the bacteria that live within us and those that live within the very different digestive systems of ruminants take their turns and break the stuff down as best they can. When they can't break it down, as is often the case with beans and a few other plant foods, we may even become slightly . . . musical (hence the "beans, beans, the musical fruit" song from childhood). The same thing happens to cows when they eat stuff their bodies can't digest.

What's really fun about this process is that one of the metabolic by-products of this intestino-bacterial shakedown is butyric acid, which is reabsorbed by the colon right back into our bodies. Butyric acid is a saturated fatty acid—its name comes from the Greek word for butter. Vegan or omnivore, you'll get your butter one way or another. (Nanny-nanny boo-boo, your bacteria is buttering you!)

Understanding, then, that creature foods are digestible and more nutrient-dense than plants and that they possess more bang for the caloric buck—especially when packaged with their natural fats and nutrients and cooked for maximum digestibility—we reach the most beloved antiomnivore argument of all: that it's downright cruel, from an animal welfare standpoint and an environmental perspective, to eat animals.

Don't be cruel
(or, veganism: I get it)

....

I really do get it.

People stop eating meat for a variety of reasons (I did once, too), and environmentalism and cruelty-free living represent the best of intentions. It is, as Miracle Max would say, a very noble cause. It's also socially rewarded: We perceive the meat-free to be staunch ideological heroes and healthy-living icons. Moreover, we just like to think that nothing had to die to fill our dinner plates.

Unfortunately, none of this stands up to scrutiny.

We're not omnivores because we're cruel, kill-happy executioners. We're omnivores by design. We're designed to use the nutrients from creatures more effectively than the nutrients from plants, just as herbivores use the nutrients in plants more effectively than the nutrients in animals. (You can't make a carnivore out of an herbivore any more than you can make an herbivore out of an omnivore.)

This book is, at its core, about examining our modern attitudes toward food and analyzing why we've strayed so far from our traditional, ancestral diet. This is where science, history, and critical thinking converge (along with movie quotes and dated pop culture references, of course). I've talked about how we need the nutrients that are packaged with creature protein. I've talked about how our bodies process the foods we eat. Now it's time to talk about what animals have actually meant to humans throughout history, why cruelty-free is a fallacy, why environmentalism is well served by omnivorism, and why eating creatures can help us reconnect with our nourishment in a way we once knew but have somehow forgotten.

Thanks to Kellogg, the anti–animal foods activist, and Keys, the antifat crusader—both of whom made us afraid of real, natural food—as well as the crop oil industry, which demonized animal fats while selling their industrial by-products to the burgeoning factory-farming industry, we've spent the last hundred years becoming progressively more disconnected from the animals that used to mean more to us than just meat.

Chicks, man. (And pigs. And cows. And other things with faces and feelings.)

Yes, creatures mean nutrition. But to a clued-in omnivore (or, like, any human being who lived prior to the dawn of the supermarket culture), they also mean enrichment, stability, soil fertility, and year-round food. Backyard chickens mean eggs, meat, broth, and compost, all for the small price of keeping these birds safe and well fed with nutrition as simple as the bugs from your yard. Beasts of burden can provide everything from food to tillage to transportation to protective clothing, as well as the heavy hooves to help recycle their own you-know-what back into the soil. Some cultures even burn dung for winter warmth.

Piggy banks are appropriate places to keep our savings, as British farmer and author Simon Fairlie points out, because they represent the role of the pig in history: A pig in the homestead meant zero waste and added wealth, because good old Babe delighted in eating whatever food humans couldn't. A pig, in return for regular meals and a safe haven from predators, provides a wealth of pork-tastic calories packed with B vitamins, vitamin D, and complete protein.

While machine-driven agriculture and factory farming seem to be our current default mode of growing food, at one time the process of obtaining calories wasn't outsourced at all. Not too long ago, animals were critical to the success of both the homestead and the entire community. Even as forests were cleared for crops to make more calories available to feed more people, animals still served as safeguards against hunger and even economic downturn. How? When crops fail, creatures often survive, and animals can turn foliage inedible to humans into nutritious, highly digestible food (and highly usable fertilizer).

The importance of animals to a society's economic well-being has led to their incorporation into several religious systems. For those who point to Buddhist ethics of nonviolence or the Hindu "sacred cow" as a rationale for vegetarianism, there is a pervasive feeling that eating meat leads to spiritual self-destruction. Yet these taboos are up for debate. For instance, scholars generally agree that, although Buddhists are against violence, their doctrine does not prohibit eating meat not killed by the human hand. A cow that died of natural causes could be consumed without violating religious code.

As is the case with many cultural taboos, Hindus began regarding the cow as sacred not due to religious conviction alone but also due to codes of conduct that became religious doctrine as their culture blended with that of Buddhists. These codes also arose out of concern for waning resources and ecological constraints. From the smallest tribe to the largest sect, religious codes don't necessarily come from "on high." Many of them originate out of environmental or economic necessity rather than spiritual mandate. Often, they represent the institutionalization of gratitude and respect for a particular resource or provision and are intended to have an impact on behavior toward it on a broad scale.

These secular origins don't mean that the values themselves are spiritually worthless, however. It simply means that theology often arises out of nonreligious necessity. We tend to forget this because we have *all* the provisions, *all* the time. We rarely feel a need to conserve or protect an important resource through religion. We forget this becau[se] right now, most of us are really freaking lucky.

Reverence for a particular animal doesn't always result in a religious taboo against consuming it, of course. The first time I saw *Dances with Wolves*—back when televisions weren't flat and Kevin Costner was better able to teach me cultural lessons than my American history classes—I realized that animals could be so greatly revered that the opportunity to hunt them, eat them, and use their hides and bones was considered a sacred, spiritual event. The ritualistic and religious importance of creatures as food is ingrained in traditional cultures across the globe—at least in those whose nourishment is neither guaranteed nor housed in cute, colorful rows at the local market. As cultural anthropologist Richard Nelson wrote, "The supermarket is an agent of our forgetfulness."

And, as Kevin Costner learned, as much as the kill is of paramount importance, to waste a single part of an animal is the ultimate act of greed. (I could write a whole book called *Things I've Learned from Kevin Costner.*) Nelson recounts food-finding expeditions with native Koyukon hunters in Alaska as experiences of great spiritual significance:

> *Traveling with Koyukon hunters, I came to understand that... the creature gives itself to a person who has honored and respected others of its kind. Koyukon villagers are mindful that they move in a world filled with power far greater than their own; power that allows no place for arrogance, waste, indifference, or disregard.*

Modern-day, indiscriminate opposition to creatures as food is often a response not to traditional hunters like the Koyukon but to the horrors of factory farming and the problems with industrial meat. Anyone who has watched the film *Food, Inc.* knows the feeling of shock and revulsion that comes with witnessing the horrors of today's industrial feedlots, but it's a huge mistake to confuse these practices—which are conducted for maximum profit without regard for

on, animal welfare, or environmental health—
ghtful omnivorism I advocate, which is focused
ent, nose-to-tail eating, appreciation of the ani-
(or, as farmer and author Joel Salatin would call
it, "the pig-ness of the pig"), and the health of the topsoil that
makes it all possible.

The truth is, a plant grown in a constant shower of pesticides, in nutrient-stripped soil supplemented with artificial
fertilizers, is no healthier than an animal raised in an unnatural environment on food it wasn't meant to eat, supplemented with a laundry list of antibiotics and other pharmaceuticals. How we treat our food—plant or animal—matters.
When we do our best to honor it by harnessing natural processes rather than attempting to override them, we have the
extraordinary effect of fostering a nutrient-filled, low-waste
food web.

Ruminants like cows and bison are made to eat grass,
not corn, soy, or candy wrappers, and they're made to live
on pasture and rangeland. They're supposed to poop non-
toxic meadow muffins, which they then stomp into the grass,
returning nutrients to the soil. Monogastrics like pigs and
chickens aren't vegetarians; they're omnivores, meant to live
outside in woods or pasture while doing the same doo-doo
dance. Animals living this way are healthy, and when they're
slaughtered for meat, they become healthy food for apprecia-
tive omnivores.

When animals eat the wrong food and live in the wrong
environment, however, they become the wrong food for us,
too. Corn-fed cows, for example, are deficient in the amino
acid tryptophan. Their meat ends up being a vehicle for anti-
biotic resistance and a carrier for exogenous hormones and
pathogens, such as mad cow disease and foot-and-mouth disease, which are products of unscrupulous feedlot industry
practices in the first place. Factory farms can even become
breeding grounds for *E. coli*, though that bacteria has also

contaminated both factory-farmed turkey and supermarket spinach (the problems of a centralized, industrial food system aren't specific to animals). In a factory farm, poop is washed into waste pits using pumped-in water, creating a mix that enables bacteria to thrive and produce the methane gas that livestock is often blamed for. It's not natural, it's not nice, and I don't support it.

Oh, and also: It stinks. Try driving across Kansas, my home state, and you'll catch your fill of feedlot whiffs. When these animals are being raised right, however, there's no smell but nature—because there's nothing there but grass, animals, rich soil, and sunshine.

"Doing it right" brings me to the topic of hunting, which, like gathering, is a long-established means of securing nourishment from nature. There's a reason "hunting and gathering" is, for all intents and purposes, a single activity: because relying on just one, rather than a mix of both, is impractical in the wild (that's the underlying truth of omnivorism). Opposition to hunting is, at the core, a symptom of our extreme privilege and disconnection from the skills needed for survival, the skills that many traditional cultures—some living in remote corners of the world—still employ with a "waste not, want not" ethos.

According to a survey of American attitudes toward nature, those who are most against hunting generally understand and experience nature the least. They tend to be women living in large cities who have no involvement with animals or the outdoors (a description that fit me to a T during my vegan dabble-days). It may seem counterintuitive, but some of the people with the greatest knowledge of and appreciation for nature are hunters. These "nature hunters," as they were termed in the survey, hunt as a means of engaging with the process of life, death, and subsistence with an attitude of reverence and respect. It's the folks who don't often engage with nature one-on-one who tend to miss the point. They're far enough removed from the reality of death that they may see it only on the screen at the local movie theater—certainly not on their dinner plates.

Some might say that we should be grateful that our modern lives have freed us from having to kill our own food, but from a holistic perspective—one that takes into account the desire to practice respectful stewardship of nature rather than circumventing it or beating it into submission—it's part of the deal.

And guess what? I'm no self-sufficiency guru. I'm an amateur homesteader with a flock of chickens, a few goats, and a failed garden. I admit it: I don't know how to hunt, and I've never field-dressed a deer. Learning to hunt and process my own food is certainly on my bucket list, but for some reason it's harder to hunt and fish legally than it is to buy the carcass of a mistreated, antibiotic-laden animal from the local supermarket. The next best thing is to support local, ethical, pasture-based producers of traditional foods like beef, bison, pork, and poultry—an excellent alternative to do-it-yourself. Wild food and ethically raised food alike are never given hormones or antibiotics; however, every creature has hormones in it. That's why it's illegal to label a meat "hormone-free," but "no added hormones" is allowed.

Guess why this isn't a strike against animal foods? Because plants have hormones, too. Or at least they have substances similar to hormones that can drive our own natural hormones cray-zay. (More on that in chapter 3.)

All this considered, eating wild-caught or properly raised creatures still involves killing something with a mother and a face and a Disney movie dedicated to its hilarious, anthropomorphic exploits, and that's the most difficult part. Even if we accept that animals are more nutritious than plants, that we're meant to digest them, and that history and biology have carved out our omnivorous ecological niche, it's sometimes still difficult to envision eating a big ol' pot of Bambi stew.

Why cruelty-free is a fallacy

Unfortunately, many of us are educated about animals by the entertainment industry, and through that lens we acquire an image of nature that is wildly and tragically inaccurate. It's an image with a rosy filter, one that ignores the fact that nature itself is, and always has been, engaged in a cycle of life and death—a cycle that seems cruel and violent rather than innate and natural when we're raised on Disney instead of Discovery.

Nelson puts it this way:

> *If the characters in Bambi's world are distortions of real animals, the forest they inhabit has almost nothing in common with an actual environment and almost totally lacks a sense for ecological relationships. Rabbits, mice, and grouse live harmoniously with carnivores like skunks, raccoons, and great horned owls. Herbivores take an occasional nibble, but predators never eat.*

This is not reality. In fact, *Honey, I Shrunk the Kids* is more realistic in its honesty about the perils of living in the wild (although, in this case, the "wildlife" is very small and the "wild" is the Szalinskis' backyard).

In nature, creatures kill and eat one another. From the top of the food chain to the bottom, something, somewhere, is being eaten or used by something else. For us to attribute feelings and sentience only to humans or large creatures commonly farmed for food is convenient but hypocritical. Organisms from ants to bees to mice have been found to have the ability to feel, cooperate, and form relationships, and not eating meat doesn't save these less frequently eaten creatures: Any of them can be killed off in the cultivation of beans, rice, corn, and chlorella. Just because we're not chewing on it doesn't mean it didn't suffer on our behalf, although keeping it out of our mouths also keeps it out of sight and out of mind.

Living, eating, and dying are intrinsic parts of a natural design that is inherently beautiful, but our inability to accept that cycle causes fear and stimulates our impulse to turn away from it entirely, abdicating both our place in it and our responsibility to it. And if we allow the wild animal its inborn capacity to kill while insisting that we humans are somehow different—whether because of our ecological position or our ability to reason—we don't give full credence to what it takes to get any type of food to the table.

Forests, with their native wildlife and natural biodiversity, are cleared to make room for bananas, citrus, coffee, and avocados. Sustaining crop fields and agricultural operations requires us to hunt or remove from the land large, crop-loving animals like deer. The cotton clothes we wear are saturated with pesticides that decimate living things. Shrews, moles, rabbits, gophers, and sweet little field mice are plowed over, displaced, or killed in the process of growing food and clothing for vegans, vegetarians, and omnivores alike.

Some dude named Robert Burns, who felt *reeeeal* bad about running over one of these little buggers with his plow, wrote a whole poem about the field mouse in which he was happy to share a bite of corn with the little thing. These days, we don't like sharing; we prefer to use anticoagulant rodenticides to eradicate the pests that dare invade our agricultural system. And we're definitely not writing poems about them anymore. They're lucky if they get a limerick.

Beyond field mice are hundreds of millions of bacteria, scads of protozoa, and countless beetles, spiders, crickets, earthworms, and other ugly, nonfurry beings that are killed in the growth, development, and production of every vegetable we eat, whether organic or conventional, whether from large-scale operations, local farmers, or backyard gardens. The sheer act of picking and washing something puts an end to countless organisms. Eating a plant, then, might leave one's hands no cleaner than eating pasture-raised pork.

Even plants themselves possess a certain type of sentience in that they are able to sense, respond, develop, and feel in ways we're just beginning to understand. "Plants like the burr cucumber," says plant biologist Daniel Chamovitz, "are up to ten times more sensitive than we are when it comes to touch."

In our world, where food is in constant supply, we can choose what is food and what is forbidden. We can anthropo-morphize animals yet wax anthropocentric about our own existence, choosing comfort over cooperation. If an idea like hunting disgusts us, by no means will we force ourselves to do it, because our survival does not depend on it. We have grocery stores and others who do the hunting (and growing and picking and plucking) for us. But that's not the way things work when we're stripped of developed-world conveniences. All organisms must eat. All life ends in death, and we must try to understand and respond to that fact rather than deny, avoid, or ignore it.

If we truly believe that no living thing should have to die for our dinner, we shouldn't eat at all. If we truly believe that all life deserves equal respect, why not equalize ourselves by embracing the elegant fact that we are all, as Nelson writes, "driven by the same hungers that motivate any other crea-ture—the squirrel in the forest, the vole in the meadow, the bear on the mountainside, the deer in the valley"?

We can accept the natural cycle of life and death on this planet, as well as our role and responsibility at the top of the food chain, by keeping in mind that our dust will one day nourish another wave of plants, then animals. We can choose to be responsible stewards of creatures, plants, and the soil so that death isn't outsourced for the sake of our emotional comfort.

But that can feel unfair and inconvenient. It requires us to work for our food and accept the reality that existing *with nature* means existing *in nature* to the best of our ability. This is as difficult for an omnivore who has never hunted as it is for a vegan who has never had a garden. But trust me:

Despite the inconvenience of bookmarking a whole new set of recipe blogs, and despite the fact that this whole shebang is only now just gaining some hoity-toity high ground, you want to get in on the ground floor of this one. Anthronutritional-Sustainable-Food-Webism is totally the next big thing.

"There is only one kind of life, shared equally, identically, and universally among the earth's organisms," says Nelson. "We pass life back and forth—the fire that burns inside us all—creating a spectacular network of interdependence."

The eco-argument: The final straw

Simon Fairlie debunks most of the environmental arguments against raising animals for food in his book *Meat: A Benign Extravagance*. Claims that cow farts pollute and generate suffocating amounts of greenhouse gases and that cows themselves steal a disproportionate amount of water and resources are lacking at best and completely falsified at worst. Factory farming isn't innocent, and neither is crop oil monoculture, but I advocate neither; and Fairlie proves that pastured animal production is sustainable, environmentally sound, and nutritionally upright in terms of bioavailable calories and nutrition.

"Monoculture does not exist in nature, nor does waste, for whatever is waste to one species is food or habitat to another," Fairlie says. Harnessing this truth in human food production is called *permaculture,* and it does not involve the "fossil-fuel-dependent industrial farming system" or chemical agriculture.

It's no surprise that not all vegans are happy with the figures Fairlie uncovers, because, as Nelson states, "an animal rights activist is not an environmentalist." And while many animal rights activists protest factory farms, we Anthronutritional-Sustainable-Food-Webists lodge our votes against industrial farming by spending our money on their true opposition: not plants, but small, decentralized, integrated farms that are slowly but surely showing the world that factory farms are as rotten as they are nutritionally bankrupt. Some of us might even hunt a deer or two.

Animals thrive on land not suitable for crops, and the CIA's *2007 World Factbook* states that "only about 20 percent of the land in the U.S. can be cultivated for crops, but 26 percent can be used to pasture livestock." Animals pastured on nonarable land pull "otherwise inaccessible nutrients" into the food web.

We can get more nutritious calories in a sustainable, renewable fashion by opting for properly raised animal nutrition in addition to any plants we might eat. Creatures don't need to eat corn or soy, nor do we need to "feed the world" with the products of industrial agriculture.

The human-animal food relationship dates back many thousands of years, and only recently have we deemed it acceptable to keep our animals in festering conditions with plans to use whatever part is most desired in the moment while ignoring the rest. (Chicken breast is attached to *something,* even if we don't want to buy it that way.) In her book *Deep Nutrition,* physician Cate Shanahan affirms my affinity for nose-to-tail eating, stating that our bodies became used to whole-animal nutrition over the course of thousands of years, and for that reason we function best on the nutrition from animals, including their "bones, joints, and organs."

Euuuuuuuwww, right? Actually, it's all pretty dang tasty once you get into it. The argument that "just because something *feels* impossible doesn't mean we shouldn't try"—which I have heard from vegans in response to my argument that it is impossible to live outside the food chain—also applies to the concept of taking responsibility for our own nourishment, from beginning to end and from top to tail.

So here's the bottom line, and it's pretty simple: We can lessen our impact on the world and its resources while maintaining our own long-term health by choosing properly raised animal foods. We need less of those foods to thrive, and if the animals are raised right, we use less industrial intervention to get them from farm to table. Our plates might look different, but fewer bites doesn't have to mean fewer calories or less nourishment. Eating local foods and nose-to-tail is a pretty dang decent sign of respect for our food, for our own bodies, and for our environment.

So what to do?

Kick around the idea of hunting, supporting your local pasture-based farmer, or even keeping a few chickens of your own. The Internet's just sitting there—use it! And if you already do those things, show somebody else how to do them. Start a blog about it. Spread the word.

If you haven't had a bite of beef in decades, feel free to start slow. Visit a small farm.

You don't have to make sweeping changes immediately or feel persecuted if your choices don't align with the ideas I've outlined here. While factory-farmed meat and the products of industrial agriculture will never be the best choices for the health of our bodies or our planet, we didn't get here overnight, and not everyone can drop everything for the sake of making immediate change. But little by little, each of us can do something different.

Remember that, when it comes to right-raised creature nutrition, we can do more with less. Properly raised creature protein comes packaged with healthy fats, vitamins, and minerals, and calories are in rich supply. You may not need a giant plate to get what you need. Stuffing ourselves with plant matter for a feeling of fullness isn't the same as nourishing ourselves fully in keeping with our biology, and we can become full without the comparatively larger volume of plant food.

Get a little closer to your protein and where it comes from. If you can't visit the place where it's raised, or if the feed-lot stench stretches across city limits, you don't want what they're selling. You have the right to ask what your animal ate, and you should get clear answers. Cows eat grass. So do bison. Pigs eat whatever's outside—little animals, roots, and plant matter. Chickens eat bugs and grubs (they're not vege-tarians). The healthiest fish are wild-caught, not farmed. No-body—neither people nor animals—needs to be eating soy, corn, or canola by-products.

If it's from Tyson or Perdue, it's not for you.

....

Chapter 3

carbs

Carbohydrates make up some of the most convoluted, confusing dietary territory out there. (Actually, I just wanted to make you say *dietary territory*. Fun, no?)

Fittingly, this chapter isn't about carbs as we usually think about them. It's not about carb counts or the numbers on a nutrition label. It's about where our carbs come from and what they're built with, and why that matters more than any carb count. It's also about crops and other plants—sources of carbs that are vastly different but not respected as such in the School of Conventional Wisdom.

Carbs, crops, and plants are all tied up in one big ball of misinformation and misconceptions. We try to make eating simple by going "high-fiber" or "whole-grain" or "low-carb" so we can establish some parameters that make life a little easier. Then someone like me comes along and shoots that all to hell.

Sorry, but I'm not sorry.

Here's the truth: Everything we've been told about carbs—where they come from and which ones are healthy—is wrong. Wrong like a denim tuxedo.

What we take for granted as a healthy-lifestyle given—eatin' carbs, crops, and plants—is actually extremely murky water, and getting true clarity requires some context. The good news: Knowing your carbs, crops, and plants means a beautifully healthy body, crash-free energy, and, most important, a foolproof, highly sensitive bullshit meter. This will make you smarter and savvier than the average eater, and aren't the smart kids usually the popular ones, too?

Anyone? Bueller?

We often think of carbs in terms of the foods they come in. There are lots of carb sources out there. There are simple sugars, nectars, juices, and syrups, some of which are more refined than others. There are grains, such as rice, wheat, and corn, and the multitude of products made from them, whole grain or otherwise, from bread to pasta to granola bars. There are the carb sources we spend hours agonizing over in the supermarket, gingerly removing boxes and bags of so-called health foods and "all-natural" items from the shelf to read their labels, only to put them back because the nutritional jargon leaves us even more confused.

Don't get me started on which of those misleading labels we're reading, either. The ingredients list? The nutrition facts? The carbs or the net carbs? The marketing labels that say "whole grain" or "good source of fiber"? Ultimately, whether whole grain or otherwise, whether boxed, bagged, or splashed with marketing jargon, most of it is the same carb-rich garbage—let's call it carbage.

This applies to the common sources of carbs we see on supermarket shelves, even those we've been taught are healthy or, at the very least, not harmful—including cereal, bread, pasta, tortillas, wraps, bran muffins, buns, bagels, boxed grains, "whole" grains, bagged grains, flour, wheat, and anything made with or from the aforementioned. They are simply carbage, and despite what their labels may claim, they're not good for us. (Please don't be mad at me. Be mad at the manufacturers.)

Does all the carbage confusion seem overwhelming? I promise, making great choices is far simpler than you might think. In fact, it's elegantly simple: Carbohydrates from whole fruits and vegetables (not their premade juices or syrups or crystals, which are just processed versions of the real thing) are the only carb sources we need to be healthy.

Good? Good. Now I'll go ahead and muddy up the waters with lots more words.

This book is all about information and, of course, busting the BS. And no BS-busting party is complete without a rundown of what carbs, crops, and plants in general are really all about, the lies we've been told, how we came to believe them, and how we can set things right.

By the way, before we get started: This chapter wasn't written to prove why things like refined flour, refined sugar, high-fructose corn syrup, and the junk foods made from them are total garbage. (In case I need to say it, though: They're total garbage.) While most of us can withstand the aftereffects of the occasional pure-sugar hit—think real cane sugar in your coffee or a well-made dessert—processed junk foods often also contain trans fats and toxic industrial chemicals, which aren't safe in any amount. If you have lingering doubts about that, I can refer you to my good friend Google.

Crops and carbage

More than any other edibles on the market, with the possible exception of crop oils, carb-rich foods made from large-scale industrial agricultural crops—wheat, corn, and other grains, and even those made from cash crops like soy—have an entire Assembly of Evil behind them.

I'm not pointing fingers at the small farmers who make a living growing acres of crops on their land. I'm talking about the multibillion-dollar entities that drive the agricultural industry, strong-arming citizens and farmers who find themselves facing the choice of losing their livelihood or playing by the rules created by the megacorporations that control our industrial food supply. I'm talking about the head honchos of the crop conglomerates and the United States Congress, which continues to award them government subsidies. I'm talking about the agricultural lobby and even the higher-ups at the U.S. Department of Agriculture and the Food and Drug Administration, which have welcomed a revolving door of executives plucked straight out of agribusiness.

These are the powers that drive the market for our modern, mass-produced whole-grain breads and pastas, processed granola bars, low-fat boxed and bagged supermarket products, refined sugar, and even trendy organic sweeteners. It doesn't matter if these carb-rich crops are added to animal feed or made into the crap we've been told is healthy (or the junk we know isn't healthy at all). Almost every loaf of bread, box of pasta, box or bag of so-called health food, and package of diet-busting junk food at the grocery store is a product of the power of Big Fat Giant Agribusiness. And BFG Agribusiness is trampling the health of both our bodies and the planet under its big, dirty, genetically modified feet. And, like Pinky and the Brain and Bebop and Rocksteady, BFG Agribusiness is not acting alone.

Factory farms and industrial agriculture: Twisted sisters

We often hear about the meat and dairy lobby as if it's some kind of evil empire. And in truth, the hooves of big factory-farm conglomerates aren't clean. As I type this in a Midwestern coffee shop, I see the sad evidence of factory farming drive by again and again: half-dead chickens in tiny cages being shipped from God-knows-where to their deaths. A good stretch of highway in my home state of Kansas stinks of factory farms, which have invaded the state like Quantrill's Raiders (Kansas joke). I used to think this was normal before I realized what real food was.

But too many people think that the industrialization of food is only about animal products. While we've been steered (pun intended) toward thinking of the animal product industry as the pinnacle of cruelty and waste, much of the carb, crop, and plant industries are far more dangerous because they hide the blood on their hands—often through the noncommissioned hard work of animal rights groups and vegetarian activists who don't realize a few key things. Things like:

- The growing and harvesting of crops causes creatures of all shapes, sizes, and kinds to suffer and even die. (I talked about this in chapter 2.)

- Many plants, especially grains, aren't health foods at all. (More on that later.)

- Most crops, plants, and plant-based products in the supermarket are produced using synthetic, polluting nitrogen fertilizers that were first created with the leftover ammonium nitrate used in explosives during World War II. Yum.

These facts are all related, and it doesn't stop there: Without all the surplus synthetically fertilized crops, we'd have no fuel to fire that factory farm. (Say that five times fast.) Where else could the factory-farm feed come from? Whatever isn't made into cosmetics, plastics, high-fructose corn syrup, Tofutti, Tofurkey, soy protein isolate, or whole-grain what-have-you goes straight to the CAFO. Whether you eat of the CAFO, the HFCS, or any other by-product of the processed-food industry, you're part of the blood meal.

But you can opt out of the crazy. We'll talk about that. (The acronyms? You're stuck with them for the time being.)

Industrial agricultural crops and factory farms are inextricably intertwined. Animals are mistreated, raised unnaturally, and slaughtered on assembly lines because our precious grains, corn, and soy—the backbone of the "health food" industry—make up the feed for these operations. This feed makes the animals grow fatter and faster. That's how factory farms got started, and that's how they keep churning out animal products that are as unhealthy as the feed.

Everyone was once up in arms, and rightly so, over recombinant bovine growth hormone, or rBGH, a hormone created by Monsanto, a company responsible for many genetically modified organisms (GMOs). This synthetic hormone was given to dairy cows to increase milk production and had the side effect of making them very sick. Yet the agricultural industry has managed to distract us from the fact that their crops and carbage serve a similar function: They make livestock grow faster, increasing production for the sake of profit, while making the animals ill. These crops are grown in overworked, nutrient-stripped soil, which makes them even less nutritious, whether they are eaten by animals or people.

Repeat after me: We are what our animals eat. We are also what our plants absorb from the soil. When there's nothing in the soil, we aren't consuming nutrients, whether we eat the plant itself or the animal that ate that plant.

Here's how conventional contemporary agriculture and the growing of industrial crops damage the soil. First, it's important to understand that soil is not just dirt. It is the Earth. It imparts nutrition to every plant, every animal, and every human on the planet. Soil is composed of organic matter, nutrients, insects, worms by the millions, and microorganisms by the billions. Decaying compost, manure, the action of microorganisms, and the shedding of worm castings add nutrients to the soil; in turn, those nutrients are taken up by the plants that are able to take root and grow. Plants feed the insects and animals that provide that manure and eventually turn into compost, and the cycle continues. This process of soil enrichment and reenrichment, collectively known as *soil fertility,* is designed to occur constantly, over the course of thousands of years, with the cooperative action of all the organisms found in this amazing system. Unfortunately, it takes only a few years of intensive conventional agriculture to wipe out the fertile soil, minerals, and organisms that it took thousands of years to build.

Conventional contemporary agriculture is built on the concept of production, production, production rather than on soil fertility, which means that it falls far outside nature's soil-building time line. Soils are depleted before they can be replenished, and soil depletion means that fields must be artificially fertility-ized. These *fertilizers,* which contain nitrogen, are meant to replace the natural nitrogen "fixers" that become imbalanced in massively overworked soil: bacteria. (Nitrogen, as discussed in chapter 2, is a critical substance, but natural nitrogen is used differently than synthetic nitrogen.) Where the natural "carrying capacity" of nitrogen-fixing bacteria keeps soil nitrogen balanced, indiscriminate use of synthetic fertilizers leads to nitrogen excess and runoff, which poisons rivers and causes "dead zones"—like the one that covers as much as eight thousand miles in the Gulf of Mexico, which is fed by the Mississippi and receives its chemical runoff from industrial agriculture operations that leach industrial fertilizers and sewage into tributaries.

Pesticides, which are used in massive quantities to kill living things that might jeopardize the survival of cash crops, have the same runoff risk as synthetic fertilizers. Just as overuse of antibiotics creates antibiotic-resistant bacteria, indiscriminate pesticide use can create resistant pests. It can also kill pests' natural predators (also known as *beneficials*). Pesticide residues are left behind in the crops themselves and can be passed along to the animals and people who eat them. Herbicides, which are basically mass-scale weed killers, can also breed herbicide-resistant plants; worse yet, they poison animals and the living things—including the nitrogen fixers—within the soil. Like synthetic fertilizers and pesticides, herbicides don't stay contained in the open-air fields in which they're used: They enter our air and water.

By contrast, here's what happens when we take industrial crops and carbage out of the equation and begin using land more sustainably by allowing animals to graze on nutrient-rich pasture, eating their natural diets and adding their

ertilizer, manure, to the teeming ecosystem of the
oil:

- We don't shove by-products of the crop and carbage industries down animals' throats, disregarding what their bodies are built to eat and how they're built to eat it.

- We allow chickens to be chickens, pigs to be pigs, and cows to be cows. Then we allow humans to be humans and eat the foods we're naturally programmed to eat.

- We get nutritious, delicious meat rich in nutrients like cancer-fighting conjugated linoleic acid, which is produced only in the bodies of ruminant animals eating their natural diets, as well as omega-3 fatty acids and vitamin A.

- We allow the fields to be fertilized by the type of by-product we actually want: fresh manure. When it's not hosed into a cesspool and combined with water that allows methane-generating bacteria to thrive, poop is actually able to return to the earth and enrich it. Factory farms opt for the cesspool, which is why they stink, while grassy, rolling hills dotted with free-range cattle smell lovely, earthy, and natural.

- We establish a direct line between the food and the person eating it, cutting out the agribusiness middlemen who stand between you and your soy milk, canola oil, or granola bar. Also: Please don't eat those things.

I don't advocate factory-farmed meat any more than I advocate factory-farmed wheat, but the horrors of industrial animal production have been revealed so many times that our outrage distracts us from the true change that needs to be made. We don't need to stop eating animals altogether in favor of plants, plants, and more plants. We need to become responsible stewards of the natural world, our own biology, and the deeply ingrained cycles of life on Earth. We've got to get in touch with our food and the reality of how it is—and should be—produced.

Yet agricultural products and plants continue to get a free pass, as if their cultivation and consumption never hurt a fly. I'm calling cow patties on that. Mass-produced crops and carbage hurt animals, people, and the Earth.

It's total marketing mastery that has made nutritionally worthless crap—er, crops—a staple at the factory farm and the modern table despite its ability to harm. And so we move on to how this junk is marketed to us and why we fall for the slick tricks of the crop-vertising trade.

It's all about the advertising

Of course, advertising is important for any profit-generating product. If we do some detective work—and by "detective work" I mean "watching television"—we can start to see what companies and corporations think of us by paying attention to the commercials we're shown.

If you watch *Monday Night Football*, advertisers think you're someone who needs prostate-related medication, a space-age razor blade, or another beer. And they think you'll buy that stuff. They hedge that bet with their marketing budgets. If you watch late-night television, advertisers think you're likely to buy anything that involves an installment plan or a blanket with sleeves. (Confession: I own three Snuggies.) And no matter what you watch, advertisers think you'll believe anything you hear in a commercial, even if science or common sense dictates otherwise. They think you'll do whatever they tell you to do, and they aim to line their pockets in the process.

How do I know this? Because I'm dedicated to market research. And to watching television. And on any channel during any given show, from reality programs to prime-time sitcoms to whatever teen-angsty *Diaries* is the trend of the moment, we're being sold a crop-storm of industrial carbage that's disguised as food that's good for us.

Despite what the commercial of a happy, skinny woman walking through a field with a bowl of whole-grain cereal at sunrise would like you to believe, industrial crops aren't good for you, for animals, or for the Earth. Truth is, whether you buy into the Paleo concept or not, even modern "healthy" whole-grain products are just processed junk. Soy, the crop darling of the health food industry, isn't a health food at all. We believe these products are good for us not because they're healthy but because they're well advertised, because they have the weight of decades of dogma behind them, because the corporations that make them know exactly how to fund and manipulate medical studies to their advantage, and because at some point in the last fifty years, we forgot how to identify ingredients, trust our instincts, and use common sense when it comes to food and our health.

Processed profit products are total dietary punks. Some of the processed junk in today's supermarket, like candy and soda, is clearly garbage. Other processed junk hides behind phrases like "all-natural," "low-fat," "whole-grain," "high in fiber," and "may lower cholesterol." These products can't be trusted, despite their colorful packaging with beautiful images meant to make us associate Brand X with sunshine and nature. This is why margarine, granola bars, and other fake-nature garbage often come in green or yellow packaging. They want us to think it's from nature when, really, it would never exist without a factory.

And then there are the shameless celebrity endorsements, in which This Athlete or That Boy Band lets you know that *This company paid a truckload of cash for a half-day, half-assed acting gig.*

Few foods are marketed as aggressively as the ones made from industrial crops like wheat, corn, and soy. (Soy may not supply the same carb hit, but it's certainly part of the problem.) Profit margins are huge on these foods, and for good reason—the crops they're made from are grown cheap, they're cheap to manufacture, and they're sold at prices high enough that we can almost believe they're not acting cheap inside our bodies.

When they can get away with it, corporations market industrial crops and the products made from them as healthy. And they get away with it a lot. They've taught us to perceive certain buzzwords as synonymous with *healthy,* which is why they plaster the entire cereal aisle—which, if we're honest, is just boxes of cardboard containing sugar-laced cardboard— with the words *whole-grain* and *all-natural.* If the product is labeled *organic,* we think it's even better, even though it's just a better version of the same garbage—the lesser of two evils. We've been trained to think these words mean something profoundly good. We almost take those words as some kind of guarantee that the product is a bastion of health and wellness.

But here's the truth: All that marketing is covering up some pretty damn dangerous stuff. The bloated ad budgets of Corn-This, Big Soy, and Whole-Grain-That exist not because the products are healthy and they have a moral imperative to tell the world, but because the crops are government subsidized, the products are cheap-cheap-cheap to make, and every single one sucks in profits right along with that last piece of Big Agriculture's soul.

Amid a never-ending barrage of advertising for industrial carbage, from cereal to granola bars and everything in between, tell me: How many commercials for sweet potatoes have you seen? For turnips or broccoli? For the sustainable farm using integrated pest-management techniques?

Food that requires marketing jargon, fancy-schmancy labeling, or, worse, a cartoon spokesperson (or spokes-rabbit, or spokes-tiger, or spokes-leprechaun) isn't food. It's an edible industrial product.

To be honest, we should be suspicious of anything with a heavy ad budget behind it. Money enables corporations to control the spin and bury the flip side. Campaigns like "Beef: It's what's for dinner," and "Pork: The other white meat" were financed by factory-farming fronts attempting to sell a nutritionally and ethically inferior, crop-fed product to the masses. No small farmer who's raising pigs and cows in their natural environment and on their natural diets can afford a national ad campaign.

Here's a good rule of thumb: Widely advertised products with the muscle of large corporations behind them are generally nutritionally bankrupt and do the body no favors.

We can't escape the fact that quality matters on all fronts. We are what our animals eat, and we are what the soil imparts to the plants grown in it. In the industrial agricultural system, our animals eat unnatural food, the soil is stripped to the bone, and our plants are turned into science experiments. What does that make us?

Unhealthy. Unhappy with our bodies. Searching for answers that diet books can't give us. Seen all that before? Join the club.

Let's start putting the pieces together. Let's start asking why.

Carb-, crop-, and plant-related fibsies and outright lies are fed to us on a daily basis. What we've been taught about healthy carbs, whole grains, fiber, and other carb-related edibles since we were old enough for school lunches is far from the truth. Plants are the stealth bombers of the food world: They fly above the fray, but they can drop some major munitions on the body.

And all this crop and plant confusion is rolled up in one word: carbohydrates.

Carbohydrate confusion

Before we go any further, let's talk about an interesting issue that always pops up in the carb conversation. It never fails: A discussion of carbohydrates inevitably brings to mind

142

the ubiquitous low-carb diet. The low-carb movement is often conflated with the Paleo movement, so let's take a moment to parse out the facts.

Low-carb eating is a way to control insulin by controlling blood sugar. It's a biological fact that eating carbohydrates, whatever the source, ends in the delivery of sugar to the bloodstream in the form of glucose, which stimulates the production of insulin, and insulin has a fear-inducing repu- tation as a fat-storage hormone. While insulin's primary role is to make needed glucose available to our cells for the gen- eration of energy, it's true that any glucose not used for en- ergy can contribute to weight gain, insulin resistance, and problems with blood-sugar regulation.

Carbs in excess—and the definition of *excess* varies from person to person and food to food—can stimulate fat storage. Sometimes this means body fat; other times it means blood fat. Another word for blood fat: *triglycerides*. High triglycer- ides may signal that something is going wrong inside your body. It means that your body isn't able to handle the amount of carbohydrate you're eating. High triglycerides represent a high potential for inflammation of any kind, including the kind that affects your arteries.

Even people who can eat whatever they want and never get fat may have high triglycerides, simply because their bodies can't process all the sugar they eat. That's why "skin- ny" doesn't always equal "healthy." It's what's going on inside that matters.

Eating carbs in chronic excess can also lead to type 2 dia- betes, although the media often still blames this disease of blood-sugar regulation and insulin resistance on eating fatty foods despite the biological fact that fat intake has absolute- ly nothing to do with blood sugar or insulin. *Headsmack.* I watched countless news reports on Paula Deen's controver- sial type 2 diabetes diagnosis that blamed the disease not on grains and sugar-filled pastries but on the "fatty" fried egg, beef patty, and bacon she sandwiched between two glazed doughnuts on her cooking show. (Yes, that actually happened—the news reports *and* the doughnut burger.)

Contrary to those news reports, saturated animal fat was not the problem. (Although it's true that fats from crop oils and trans fats from partially hydrogenated crop oils, often used in the making of pastries and bread, can double up on the damage caused by crappy carbs and complicate sugar-related conditions.) The straight fact is that high triglycerides and type 2 diabetes aren't products of eating too much animal fat. Each of these modern afflictions, and many others, is a product of eating too many of the wrong carbs, too often, for too much of our lives, and of the metabolic damage that results.

Excess blood sugar in a person with a damaged metabolism may not get where it needs to go—that's called *insulin resistance*—and this can lead to chronically high blood sugar and type 2 diabetes. When we keep carbohydrate consumption at a level our individual bodies can manage, blood-sugar and insulin levels are reined in.

For many low-carbers, the goal is kicking the body into ketosis, a state in which the body burns fat in the absence of carbohydrates. But here's the rub: Energy from carbohydrate is recruited differently than energy from fat, and every single individual has unique activity patterns and energy needs. For some, low-carb is a panacea. For others, it's a nightmare.

Simply assessing, through trial-and-error, how much healthy carbohydrate makes you feel best is a great way to figure it all out. (I'll talk more about healthy carbs later in this chapter.) Because while maintaining healthy blood-sugar levels is important, doing so doesn't always require eating fewer carbs. Many active people find it difficult to maintain their activity levels without sufficient glucose from carbohydrates. Beyond that, carb intake isn't just about energy. Healthy carbohydrates also play a role in thyroid function, in the health of our connective tissue, and in the health of our gut bacteria. Plus, they're delicious.

Admittedly, when I went low-carb, I cared about absolutely none of this. I just wanted to trade some perfectly healthy curves for hard angles. (A story for another time.) And I have to admit that I wasn't smart about my low-carb strategy. I believed that because the carbohydrates in food—no matter what the source—break down into simple sugars within our bodies, removing a sweet potato from my daily rations was as important as removing sugary soda. That is so not the case. I've met too many folks whose low-carb diets, like mine, are high in artificial sweeteners and unhealthy fats, low in quality food, and very low in fun. My crazy version of the low-carb, low-fun diet: factory-farmed chicken, salad dressing filled with trans fats, vegetable oils, steamed broccoli, and six Diet Cokes each day (topped off with back-to-back spin classes, of course, and often a prepackaged low-carb snack bar for a treat).

The idea that a carb is a carb is a carb is totally false, and going low-carb without prioritizing food quality is a pitfall that won't keep you much healthier than if you'd kept sucking down the fat-free, sugar-free diet soda pop. (Yep, I said "soda pop.") Although a well-planned low-carb diet centered on whole, Paleo-friendly foods can work wonders for some people, for others, too little healthy carbohydrate can cause metabolic slowdown and utter cranky-pantsness. Paleo isn't low-carb, low-carb isn't Paleo, and low-carb isn't for everyone.

It's clear that this is a topic fraught with myths and misconceptions. Interestingly, however, one maxim of the low-carb lifestyle is quite true: We actually don't need carbohydrates to survive.

Stick with me, sweet-potato lovers.

Many low-carb advocates are quick to state that carbohydrate is the only nonessential macronutrient. They're technically correct, and this is the foundation of the low-carb movement.

It's true that we don't need carbs to live, but this should tell us more about the importance of healthy fat and protein than anything else. We would die without fat, because fat is needed to build our cells. Fat also carries fat-soluble vitamins and allows our bodies to use them, and our bodies can burn fat for energy. We would die without protein, because protein is needed to build our tissues. Protein also carries the amino acids we need for mental health, and our bodies can convert protein into carbohydrate in the form of glucose to be burned for energy if absolutely necessary. Without eating a single carb, we've got cell-building, structural integrity, and energy covered. But are we thriving?

That we can live without them doesn't mean carbs are bad, and this is where we run into some unfortunate misconceptions. We can't say all carbs are bad any more than we can say all people are bad. Just because your neighbor's doing great on a low-carb diet doesn't mean that you will, too, and it doesn't mean that a low-carb diet will bring every single person who tries it optimal health. And here's another truth: To say that we need carbs at all costs, and to fret and hem and haw about giving up grains—the carbohydrate source the U.S. government loves to recommend, subsidize, and support—is bonkers. (That's a technical term.)

Conventional wisdom tells us that carbohydrates, especially those from grains, are the body's only energy source. That's like telling a person locked in a tortilla-chip factory that his only energy source is nachos. Duh. The body will adapt to run as best it can on what it's given. (I was adapted to using nachos for fuel between 2002 and 2006. I miss college.) But just because the body can adapt to running on carbs doesn't mean that it *has* to run on carbs. Or nachos. Or whole grains.

Our bodies use carbohydrates for energy when we give them carbohydrates. When we give them healthy carbohydrates along with healthy fats and protein, that's fine and dandy. When we don't and instead expect our bodies to run on a low-fat diet based on carbage, as conventional wisdom suggests, we run into problems, especially with blood-sugar management. Blood-sugar highs and lows lead us to eat more often to keep from crashing, and this is the source of the "eat multiple small meals a day" myth: Carbage on a low-fat diet makes us that much hungrier, driving us to eat every danged two and a half hours. Eating every two and a half hours doesn't keep our metabolisms going. It keeps our bodies in a constant state of digest-without-rest and masks blood-sugar issues while we tell ourselves that food just can't keep us satisfied for many hours.

While there's nothing wrong with using healthy carbs for energy as part of a diet that also includes healthy fats and quality protein, modern supermarket carbage is always going to be dirty fuel. We'll get to that.

With fat and protein in our diet and without carbs, we wouldn't keel over or turn into pumpkins. We'd certainly miss our sweet potatoes, though. Panera might go out of business. We all might be a little cranky at first. The thyroid, joints, and gut bacteria might give a few of us the angry fist wave. But we'd be alive. We'd be fuller and more satisfied than we could be on a low-fat diet. And we'd probably be healthier than the majority of Americans, who scarf down whole grains like it's their health salvation.

I say this not because I'm a low-carb advocate or because I think we shouldn't eat carbs at all. I've just got to throw it out there so that when you're on your vision quest through the wilderness with one rucksack each of fat, protein, and carbs, and you're forced to give one rucksack to a bridge troll before you can cross the river, you'll know which bag to trade: the bag of carbohydrates.

Some may find that information more useful than others.

The rest of the time, you can feel free to eat the dang carbs. The good ones, that is.

Good carbs are not the enemy

Despite the fact that eating carbohydrates is not essential to our ability to live, love, or write Paleo books, there are many forms of carbohydrates that are totally legit. Carbs are not the enemy when they come from the right sources. Actually, the right carbs can amplify a healthy diet to sonic boom status.

The government, most nutritionists, and most doctors say that you need to eat carbs in some form or another. Usually, they're talking about grains—despite the fact that vegetables and fruits are a better source of carbohydrates, provide more bioavailable nutrients along with their carbs, and are a more appropriate source of fiber than modern grain-based supermarket carbage.

To add to their utility, healthy carbs from certain fruits and vegetables feed something very important—something that can make or break your health, your immunity, and even your ability to achieve and maintain a healthy weight. I'm talking 'bout your gut bacteria, the "good bacteria" that live in your digestive tract. You want to keep these little critters happy because they are involved in keeping you full, shoring up your immune system, ensuring that your bowels are healthy, and keeping your weight stable. (More on that when we get to fiber.)

It's not as complex as it sounds. In fact, these are simple swaps: Get your dense carbs from sweet potatoes instead of bread. Boom. Have a plantain instead of a pancake. Pow. Pile caramelized onions over your dandelion greens instead of adding croutons. Shazam.

This might feel complicated at first. It certainly demands more of us than conventional wisdom's list of "good for you" foods. We actually have to know what we're doing when we choose food. It sucks, because it's much easier to pretend that our nagging physical issues, from poor sleep to poor digestion to poor energy, have nothing to do with what we eat. It's much easier just to follow a list of rules or demonize a macronutrient, as if its exclusion holds the key to health for everyone, and call it good.

First it was fat (thanks, Ancel Keys). From there, animal protein got a bad rap. Then it was carbs (thanks, Atkins).

So what's a Real Housewife to eat? A kale and oxygen smoothie?

Actually, I'm pretty sure that *is* what they eat.

But I repeat: Carbs are *not* the enemy. They are not the enemy. They. Are. Not. The. Enemy.

As long as you choose the right carbs, that is, in the right amount for you, with a full understanding of why you're making those choices. And that's where this chapter gets really good.

There are a few things I know for certain about carbs.

We crave carbs for a reason

Strip away the supermarkets and the farmer's markets. Forget about all the people and machines and industries that exist to produce food for us. Think about being able to eat only what you can hunt and gather. While animal fat and protein keep you fit, functioning, and alive, a hit of carbs from a patch of berries provides a shot of energy that can overflow into your fat cells to provide fuel to burn in times of scarcity. This is everything you could hope for: the sweet taste of survival. And this is why we are programmed to appreciate a good carb hit.

It's more deeply ingrained than our desire to diet. It's programmed into who we are as organisms working to survive. This deep programming is why we find it so hard to resist carb-rich foods.

So not only is our modern, diet-culture desire to be thin and super-lean evolutionarily inappropriate—our bodies love to have a little extra stored away in case of scarcity or famine—but our modern access to food, especially carbs, and the modern demands on our energy (sitting, sitting, and more sitting) are as well. That's a perfect storm of diet confusion, and it explains why the world of weight loss, dieting, health, and food continues to make us all crazy.

This brings me to the second thing I know for certain about carbs.

Our modern access to carbs is unnatural, and this can cause problems

In most of the world—without greenhouses, farm machinery, and planes, trains, and automobiles to ship sweet fruits, vegetables, and grain-based carbohydrates great distances—we wouldn't have precious, carb-rich plants available at a moment's notice, any time of year. Further, without selectively breeding fruits and starchy vegetables for enhanced sweetness and size, we wouldn't have those carbs in such great proportions.

This evolutionary dissonance is our downfall when it comes to carbohydrates, and it's why we're more likely to binge on carb-rich foods than any other kind. We are programmed to gorge on carbs when they're available in nature, but for most of history and in most of the world, this was a relatively rare occurrence. Even in parts of the world where carbohydrate-rich fruits and plants grow year-round, traditional cultures had to work very hard to find and gather them. Nobody climbs a banana tree to grab snacks for their desk job or risks raiding a beehive (one of the few truly natural places to find sweetener) for honey to drizzle over their low-fat Greek yogurt.

If we modeled our carbohydrate intake after nature by respecting the fact that carbohydrates are seasonal, regional gifts that come from vegetables, fruits, and honey, and avoided processed grains, low-fat diet foods, and carbage, maybe we'd be a little less confused. Knowledge is power, right?

We suffer very little scarcity in America today. Instead, we're inundated with copious carbs even as the echo of evolution is driving us to eat as much as possible whenever we're lucky enough to find food. This is why I often say, in that sardonic way I have, that "the caveman would if he could." For thousands of years, gorging on carbs provided pleasure because it was a rare occurrence that helped us survive, not because we could do it all the time, any time, as we can today. Gorging on carbs is an evolutionary mandate rooted in the ever-looming threat of scarcity. But now, even though we've conquered scarcity, we can't override our built-in drive to gorge on anything that's even remotely sweet.

Add to that the dogma of the last fifty years, and things get even worse.

As a society, we are dead-set on viewing carbage—whether the sugary-treat kind or the low-fat diet kind or the whole-grain conventional wisdom kind—as "okay," because unlike animal protein and fat, there's no long-ingrained, time-honored, batshit-crazy mainstream dogma attached to it. Carbage doesn't contain cholesterol, it doesn't have a face or a soul, and—perhaps most important—it makes a lotta companies a lotta money.

And we like to binge on it. It's every dieter's late-night addiction, and that's not an accident. It's the result of hard work by food industry scientists to replicate and intensify our affinity for natural carb-rich foods by concentrating their addictive properties within manufactured foods. A box of crackers, a carton of low-fat ice cream (which really just means high-sugar ice cream), and half a box of granola doesn't push us off the wagon, right? We can eat them in moderation, right? We can still please the diet gods, right?

Our difficulty controlling our carbage cravings led to the development of artificial sweeteners, which enable us to indulge that impulse year-round without any caloric consequences—or so we think. But we've found again and again that we can't outsmart nature: Diet soda and artificial sweeteners cause our bodies to rebel when they don't receive the calories that are supposed to come with the carbs, and cravings simply get worse. That's a likely explanation for diet soda's association with weight gain.

So the cards are stacked against us when it comes to carbage. I have overeaten crackers, bread, and pasta—even the whole-grain kind—more times than I can count. And if we believe some diet gurus, there's absolutely no physiological reason behind that. They say that there's nothing wrong with those foods or how our bodies process them, and that we should simply count our calories and learn to eat them "in moderation." Binging on carbage is a problem of willpower and our total dearth of Gwyneth Paltrow genetics. Right?

Wrong.

Here's another whack with the information paddle: Due to our digestive landscape and the way healthy foods stimulate that satisfying feeling of fullness, it's incredibly difficult to overeat carbohydrates in their whole-food forms to the degree we can overeat processed carbs. Willpower or not, I would never care to eat ten apples, but assuming each apple is 100 calories, I could easily eat the equivalent amount of energy in five 200-calorie doughnuts or seven 140-calorie Olive Garden breadsticks. When you process food out of its original form, you process all the appetite-regulating, tummy-filling potential right out of it.

What does that tell us about what our bodies need? When we eat whole, nutrient-rich fats, complete proteins, and truly healthy carbohydrates, which balance our hunger hormones instead of whacking them out, our bodies say, *I've got all I need. I don't need more.*

When we eat carbage, including the whole-grain kind, our bodies are much more likely to say, *I'm still hungry. I'm not finding what I need. More.* Partly because our bodies can recognize real food even when our eyes can't.

It's not about willpower or moderation. It's about eating the right foods.

Even in the face of all the controversy surrounding conventional carbage, people remain skeptical about the alternative, commonsense approach of eating real, unprocessed food and ditching the rest—or, put more simply, *eating a Paleo diet.* Maybe they don't know the true story behind the foods they eat. Maybe they do and just don't want to give up their cereal, bread, and pasta, nutrition be damned. Maybe they don't know how damaging carbage "in moderation" can be to the body and to the planet. Maybe they don't know that we can get just as many carbs and just as much fiber from vegetables and fruits as we can from grains. Maybe they don't really know the difference between good carbs and bad, or why fruits and vegetables are better choices than grains and carbage. We think we know our food, but often we don't.

This brings me to the most important thing I know for certain about carbs.

Carbs are not created equal

Despite having been told since childhood that bread, grains, and crop-based foods are as important to our bodies as fruits and vegetables, the carbs within these foods, and the foods themselves, are not the same—in their chemical structures, in how they affect our bodies, or in how they should be prepared. We're about to get into all that, and it's going to take some time to uncover the truth behind the myths. For now, just know that some carbs are better than others, and learning to choose the right carbs is more than half the battle.

The chemistry of carbs

In the words of Inigo Montoya, "Let me 'splain. No. There is too much. Let me sum up."

It may take me a few thousand words, but I'll "sum up" as best I can.

To this point, I've spoken about Earth-damaging crops, the tricks of carb marketing, the low-down dirty agricultural industry, and why we're so attached to carb-rich foods, especially carbage. That's important background information, and I'm all about context. Now, though, it's time to get down to brass tacks: what carbs are at the fundamental level, how our bodies use them, what exactly makes a carb-rich food good or bad, and all the other ins and outs of carbohydrates in our modern diets.

In the strictest sense, carbs are chemical structures, just like fat and protein. These chemical structures are composed of carbon, hydrogen, and oxygen, and they play starring roles in our food. There's plenty of merit in understanding those structures. That's science, and some perverts find that science is fun.

Let's expand on that. Let's expand on it like my waistline on funnel cakes.

In order to burn carbohydrates, the body must first break those carbs free of the foods they're in, and then break them down again, converting them into glucose. Glucose is the most basic carbohydrate possible—a monosaccharide—and the one and only form of carbohydrate our cells can use. Once the breaking-down process is complete, glucose enters the bloodstream. Depending on how much glucose hits our bloodstream at a given moment, we may feel totally normal, or we may feel a blood-sugar spike followed by a sudden crash, a sign that our personal carb intake or something else in our diet, like the level of healthy fat or protein, needs tweaking. A rise in blood sugar stimulates the pancreas to release insulin. Insulin shuttles the glucose to the cells, where it's used in the generation of energy.

This sounds simple. It's not.

Carbohydrates, with the exception of fiber, are all destined to be delivered to the bloodstream as glucose. Despite their shared destiny, however, not all carbs are the same. The effect of carbs on blood sugar depends on the food they're in. Some carbs, like those from sugars and syrups, require very little digestion and are absorbed quickly, hitting the bloodstream fast and hard. Others, like those within sweet potatoes, hit the bloodstream more slowly and steadily thanks to the amount of time a sweet potato takes to work its way through the digestive system. This keeps blood sugar on a more even keel.

While glucose is the monosaccharide that our cells can use, you may have heard of a couple others: galactose, which is found in lactose, a milk sugar; and fructose, the sweetest of all natural sugars, which is found in nature within fruits and honey and in the laboratory within the manufactured sweetener high-fructose corn syrup. Both galactose and fructose must be converted to glucose by the liver before being released to the bloodstream—an extra step in the process that is unique to those monosaccharides.

While the extra step of converting these sugars is part of the liver's job—a job it's well equipped to do—the constant barrage of fructose from unnatural, modern processed foods, like soda and carbage, can overburden the liver. The liver is a critical organ that needs to focus not on the processed-food follies but on doing things like packaging and eliminating toxins, disabling dangerous substances, maintaining healthy cholesterol production, and filtering bodily and environmental pollutants. This is why fructose in large amounts, especially from refined foods, soda, and high-fructose corn syrup, may contribute to modern health issues like obesity, diabetes, and heart disease. An overburdened liver that's always managing the constant assault of fructose-filled processed foods can compromise the health of the entire body. This is unlikely to become a problem within a real-food lifestyle (unless you're living on fruit and fruit alone), which is why I don't tend to freak out over naturally occurring fructose, but those living on soda and carbage are cruisin' for a hepatic bruisin'.

Carbohydrates end up as the monosaccharide glucose within our bodies, but carbohydrates in foods usually start out as disaccharides, oligosaccharides, or polysaccharides. These are carbohydrate molecules made up of multiple chemically bonded monosaccharides that are eventually disassembled within our bodies by digestive enzymes and converted into glucose. If there are two chemically bonded monosaccharides in one unit of carbohydrate, the unit is called a *disaccharide;* if there are between three and ten, it's an *oligosaccharide;* if there are more than that, it's a *polysaccharide.*

Most of the pure sugars and syrups we eat are composed of disaccharides. The most common disaccharide is sucrose, which is a unit of glucose bonded to fructose. Sucrose is found in fruits and vegetables (where it is surrounded by fiber and other nutrients), as well as in simple table sugar and high-fructose corn syrup, which is most famous for its fructose content but is actually a manufactured disaccharide of glucose bonded to fructose. Lactose is a disaccharide built from the bond of glucose and galactose and is found in milk; the disaccharide maltose, which is a bond of two glucose molecules that results from the breakdown of starch, is found in malt, which is found in beer. You probably don't need to know that stuff. I'm just showing off at this point.

Oligosaccharides are unique in that the human body doesn't produce an enzyme that can break them down, so the job falls to the bacteria that live in the colon. This can be a good thing, as we'll talk about when we get to fiber, but it can also be a very noisy thing. Bacteria can generate gas when tasked with the breakdown of oligosaccharides, which is why beans and cruciferous veggies—rich sources of oligosaccharides—have earned certain nicknames: Beans are the "musical fruit," and crucifers are also known as "crucifarts." (Actually, I think I just made that one up. And I suddenly have the urge to rewatch *Blazing Saddles.* Anyone?)

Wheat also contains oligosaccharides. So does this mean cauliflower, wheat, and beans are nutritionally equivalent? As Vizzini would say: *not remotely.* A carb is not a carb is not a carb, remember? While cauliflower is perfectly safe and nutritious in its natural state, wheat comes along with junk like gluten, lectins, and phytic acid, and those nutritional merit badges (sarcasm) are often baked into carbage replete with even more highly processed ingredients like crop oils. Blech. Beans, which can pack an unreasonable blood-sugar punch that's not backed up by ample nutrition, become digestible only after careful preparation (I'll talk about that later).

Polysaccharides, built from long chains of ten or more monosaccharides, are found in a vast array of plants: grains, beans, some fruits, starchy vegetables, and some nonstarchy vegetables like peppers and leafy greens. The polysaccharide category includes starch, which we can digest, fiber, and something called *resistant starch* (which I consider an honorary fiber), neither of which we can digest but which can still impact our health.

Starch, which is found in highest proportion in grains, beans, some fruits like plantains and bananas, and veggies like potatoes, sweet potatoes, and other roots and tubers, is broken down by digestive enzymes and delivered to the cells as glucose, just like all other digestible carbohydrates. While many people fear starchy food because they believe it has "too many carbs," that's a symptom of our carb-fearing culture more than anything. A food doesn't have to have a lot of carbs per serving to contain starch. A carb-dense starchy food, as long as it's a nutrient-dense one, can be a darn efficient way to get healthy energy. When we talk about antinutrients, it'll become clear why some starchy foods are fabulous and others are bottom-rung rubbish.

Foods high in starch are also known as complex carbohydrates. This is where things get interesting. And, also, extremely dumb.

What is a complex carbohydrate, anyway?

According to the U.S. Department of Agriculture's MyPlate dietary recommendations, grains, beans, fruits, and vegetables—all sources of carbs, and most also sources of starch—all fall into different food groups. However, the

2010 Dietary Guidelines for Americans, issued jointly by the Department of Agriculture and the Department of Health and Human Services, notes that these same foods also fall under the single umbrella of complex carbohydrates.

Here's how my behavior, for many years, reflected this awkward carb categorization: When it was convenient, I'd treat the carbage I loved eating as its own government-endorsed food group. I lamented the dangers of eliminating a whole food group as an argument against giving them up (even though I've given up animal products, fat, and even carbohydrates during various phases when I was exploring veganism, conventional wisdomism, and Atkinsism). But when it suited me, I'd do the exact opposite: I'd consider grains to be part of the same group as vegetables and fruits, as if they were interchangeable and consuming whole-grain pasta instead of summer squash was A-OK, simply because they're all sources of complex carbohydrates. Why did I do that?

Because I'd do anything to rationalize my grain addiction, that's why.

Any rationale for needing grains is actually just an excuse for wanting them, nutrition be damned. It was tough for me to imagine a life without wheat bread or pasta. But just because we like that stuff doesn't mean it's good for us. Just because we've always eaten that stuff doesn't mean we need to keep on eating it. No matter why we once thought we needed carbs from grains, pasta, bread, or anything out of a box or a bag, whether processed or whole, we were wrong. We just didn't know what we were eating.

So what are these foods really about? What defines them—their polysaccharides, their "food group," their complexity? What does it all mean?

Not much, if you ask me. Because none of those things take into account their nutritional value.

For years, we've regarded the carbohydrate-rich foods we eat as either "bad" or "good" based on whether they are labeled simple or complex. Simple carb-rich foods are the ones containing mono- and disaccharides—simple sugars—which, given their highly refined nature and their ability to cause massive blood-sugar spikes, are worthy of wariness. The complex carbs category, however—made up of foods containing polysaccharides—is highly convoluted. These foods are spread across at least three food groups in one set of guidelines and compressed into just one category in another, giving us the impression that they're all equally worthy. They're not.

Here's the problem: Some of these MyPlate-approved complex carbohydrates are simply junk passing as jewels. They're carbage that had the good fortune of being assigned to the cool carbs'—er, kids'—table.

So I asked myself: Where did we get the notion to lump 'em all together in the first place? And guess what I found out: A politician did it. Surprise!

Oh, those politicians. Always talking about crap—and crops—they don't understand. Unfortunately, unlike politicians, when I talk about crap I don't understand, I don't get the chance to turn that crap into officially recognized government policy.

In 1968, Senator George McGovern was appointed chair of the Select Committee on Nutrition and Human Needs, an appointment whose tentacles wiggled their way through the next forty years of nutrition policy. After spending nearly a decade working to expand food assistance programs, this committee shifted its focus to institutionalizing what science writer Gary Taubes calls "a grab bag of ambiguous studies and speculation" about the dangers of animal products, saturated fat, and cholesterol, as well as evangelizing the merits of a low-fat diet rich in grains, with a 1977 document titled "Dietary Goals for the United States."

McGovern, who took his cues from Nathan Pritikin, a famous low-fat-diet doctor with whom he'd briefly worked, lumped fruits, vegetables, and whole grains together in "Dietary Goals" as *complex carbohydrates,* a term McGovern coined to make the basic distinction between simple sugar and, well, everything else. It's a term we still use today, and we're still struggling with the impact of the muddled distinctions between crops, grains, grain products, beans, fruits, and vegetables and how they truly impact health.

Complex is right.

The way we think about carbs, crops, grains, grain products, beans, fruits, and vegetables has been spoon-fed to us by our government and large-industry interests for decades. When it comes to nutrition, our education system has perpetuated bad science without question. These powers-that-be had their chance to shape America's health for the better, and if the last few decades of health disasters are any indication, they failed. Miserably.

There's nothing special about America's favorite crop-based complex carbohydrates—grains and grain products—that warrants their classification in the same group as fruits and vegetables. There's also nothing so magical about them that they should be given their own food group (unless we create a new food group: worthless foods; eat zero servings daily). In fact, they belong at the bottom of the nutrition barrel. Whether they're whole or not, grain products are far more processed than fruits and veggies could ever be. It takes a lot of fertilizing, pesticide-ing, herbicide-ing, conveyor-belting, silo-storing, stoning, scouring, grinding, cracking, sieving, and fortifying to bring a loaf of bread, a granola bar, or a box of whole-grain pasta from field to supermarket. And many grain products are susceptible to contamination: Mass-cultivated rice has tested positive for arsenic, and stored corn is highly susceptible to aflatoxin—the same poison given to Campbell's rats.

But it's not just the processing that makes processed, crop-based, carb-rich foods unhealthy. It's also the other stuff that comes along with them.

What comes with your carbs?

Remember our talk about the science of carbs and how carbs in the strictest sense are chemical structures that play starring roles in our food?

Our bodies absorb the carbohydrates we eat and use them for energy. That's good, right? Eat carb, burn carb, right? No heart disease from fat (snark), no cancer from protein (snicker); just clean-burnin' plant nutrition. And plenty of fiber to boot!

Clearly, it's more complicated than that. When we talk about fat, protein, and carb in the everyday sense, we're usually talking about much more than the chemical structures themselves. That's why this whole discussion of crops, carbs, and plants matters in the first place. The fat, protein, and carb in our food are never just those chemical structures alone. Beef contains protein, but it's not only protein. Avocado contains fat, but it's not only fat. Carb sources from grains to vegetables contain carbs, but they're not only carbs. They come along with a range of other things that can help or heal, harm or benefit. Food is *not* simple. It's beautifully complex, and it's one of the few things in life worth taking the time to truly understand, right up there with the Constitution and that show with the island and the Smoke Monster and Matthew Fox.

The final test of the healthfulness of the carbs and carb-rich foods we eat is the stuff that comes along with them. And crops—especially grains—come with some serious gunk.

Grains, gluten, and gunk

The way different types of foods break down in the body is a lesson in how every molecule matters. Every part of everything we eat interacts with our bodies. Digestive enzymes, organs, hormones, and bacteria process what we eat, whether dangerous or nutritious; food helps, heals, or causes damage; and it is then passed out of the body or delivered to its final cellular destination. While carbohydrates in vegetables and fruits are found right alongside vitamins, minerals, and fiber, the carbs in crops, especially grains, are found right alongside . . . other stuff.

Let's be real: Modern grains and the so-called health foods made from them are not "whole" foods the way an apple, a sweet potato, or a strawberry is. They are processed foods, often containing crop oils and even trans fats, refined sugars, and preservatives. They contain no healthy fats and nothing in its whole, unrefined state. This is an open secret—the manufacturers don't broadcast the information, but it's right there on the label.

Yet there's another way grains cause problems. They contain compounds meant to protect the grain itself: defense mechanisms called *lectins* and *phytic acid*. Lectins are like natural pesticides—toxic compounds meant to deter would-be meal-makers, like bugs and small animals. Phytic acid is a substance within plant seeds that protects the nutrients they need to reproduce. Phytic acid binds to minerals like zinc, calcium, iron, and magnesium. It's like a little nutrient hoarder, and it doesn't like to share. Because they affect how we absorb nutrients, these defense mechanisms are sometimes known as *antinutrients*.

While lectins and phytic acid are found in many living things, including many of the foods we Paleo folk enjoy—such as nuts, seeds, and even vegetables—crops like grains, beans, and legumes (including soy) are our most concentrated sources of highly biologically active phytic acid and lectins. Grains, beans, legumes, and even the edible part of nuts are *all* actually seeds, although we call them by other names, and seeds are where these compounds are most concentrated. Why? Because seeds are the plant's reproductive force. Without legs to run, claws to scratch, or teeth to bite, plants have to protect their ability to survive through chemical means. Other seeds possess antipredation compounds as well, although this applies mostly to seeds we don't eat, so it's not such a big deal—apple seeds, peach pits, and apricot kernels all contain a cyanide compound that serves the same protective purpose.

Lectins and phytic acid are the most common plant defenses, but there are others as well. An enzyme called *myrosinase* accounts for some of the bitterness in many vegetables (bitterness is another defense mechanism), and the goitrogens in crucifers and soy may compromise thyroid function. Remember how statin drugs are derived? They're produced from a fungus whose natural defenses cripple cholesterol production.

In small amounts and as part of a varied diet, the defense mechanisms in fruits and vegetables won't impact the human body to the same degree as those from grains, beans, or soy. However, as they say, the poison is in the dose—and when it comes to the safety of an all-vegetable diet replete with thrice-daily smoothies composed of several pounds of kale, I can't really comment. (That's a joke.)

Many fruits and vegetables are biologically designed with synergistic rather than wholly defensive survival mechanisms: Their sweet flesh entices us to chow down, and, with any luck, we swallow their antinutrient-rich seeds intact and pass them out whole with ample fertilizer to allow those seeds to grow wherever they're deposited. Nature's plan works; it's how I ended up with a bevy of mulberry trees along my homestead fence line. Birds ate mulberries and distributed the seeds as they lounged on the wire. Nature is smart. Humans? Not so much sometimes.

Grains, in particular, are of most concern when it comes to defense mechanisms, because they're the source of half the world's calories. In grain-based foods, these defense mechanisms are highly concentrated, enabling the effects of these compounds to be—well—compounded.

In human nutrition, the impact of phytic acid and lectins is just beginning to be explored.

Though the immediate effects of eating something rich in phytic acid or lectins may not be apparent, long-term ingestion of foods rich in those compounds can certainly have consequences, especially in a body already stressed from poor nutrition. Lectins do their dirty work on the digestive system. They can damage gut flora, which are critical modulators of the immune system. They can also damage the gut wall, which can impact our ability to "grab" nutrients from the digestive tract and bring them into the bloodstream to be used by our cells. Phytic acid prevents minerals from being absorbed by the body. Ever had a skin problem? Could be a long-term zinc deficiency. Chronic muscle cramps? Could be a magnesium deficiency. Anemia? That's an iron deficiency. When nutrients that our cells depend on are absent for a long stretch (and how many of us have had "long stretches" of grain-based eating?), we may experience a multitude of issues.

When we're told that grains or other antinutrient-rich crops, like beans and soy, contain certain nutrients, it's important to remember that what matters isn't what the label says is in our food. It's what we're able to digest, absorb, and use. Grains, beans, and soy, and the foods made from them, may not be willing to share their nutrients with our bodies.

While many plants are filled with great nutrition, it's an undeniable truth that certain plants bite back, and some more than others. It's not their fault. It's simple biology. We're goofballs for eating them.

Another plant compound is under scrutiny for its proposed connection to everything from autoimmune disease to inflammation. It's called *gluten,* and it's a uniquely dangerous protein found in wheat, barley, rye, and other grains, as well as their derivatives, like flour and beer.

I know. My college beer-pong-playing, pizza-eating self would've shut the book right there.

Gluten-free has become a buzzword of late, but it's more than just a passing trend. Gluten can cause devastating, life-threatening symptoms in people with celiac disease, an autoimmune disease in which the small intestine is attacked by the body's own immune system in response to the ingestion of gluten. It can cause nutrient malabsorption and horrible intestinal damage.

But the disastrous effects of gluten don't end with celiac disease. New research into gluten-related disorders, led by pediatric gastroenterologist Alessio Fasano, is revealing nonceliac gluten sensitivity to be a powerful inflammatory force in the body. The medical suffix for inflammation is simply "-itis," and gluten sensitivity can manifest in any -itis, from bursitis to gingivitis, as well as autoimmune diseases, such as rheumatoid arthritis; digestive problems, including Crohn's disease; mental fog; and depression. It has even been linked to autismlike symptoms.

In the words of Joey Gladstone: Cut. It. Out.

Seriously. Cut it out. If something's going on in your body that you simply can't explain, there's a chance gluten could be involved. Don't wait for your family doctor, who is mired in patients and paperwork, to catch up with the latest in biomedical research. Just try avoiding gluten. You'll be fine— there's no such thing as a gluten deficiency.

Foods containing gluten irritate the lining of the gut and affect its permeability, even in people without celiac disease. The gut is composed of tightly aligned cells that usher nutrients into the bloodstream while keeping undesirable substances out. Gluten can act on a chemical in the body called zonulin, which causes those cells to lose their tight alignment, creating gaps where bad stuff can get through. The small intestine becomes full of more holes than Jack Nicklaus played in his career. Bad stuff, partially digested stuff, and irritating stuff gets into the bloodstream, and the body launches an immune attack to which its own tissues can fall victim. The nightmarish result for a lot of people: autoimmune disease, from multiple sclerosis to rheumatoid arthritis to Crohn's disease. For others, chronic inflammation and the other manifestations of gluten intolerance ensue. Many people find that these diseases respond favorably to a long-term gluten-free, grain-free diet.

Unfortunately, the gluten-free diet has been hijacked by big food manufacturers, spawning a new generation of processed foods. Chances are, gluten-free processed foods, just like any other processed food, contain other unhealthy junk. Gluten-free or not, if it comes in a box, bag, or package with a long ingredients list, it's not good for you.

Having steamrolled over so many beloved grain-based foods, we've also run roughshod over one of the most relentless—and most ridiculous—ongoing arguments about why we need grains in the first place. What about fiber?

The fiber factor
(or, the ins and outs of fiber)

Fiber is important, but not for the reasons we've been given, and not from the sources we think. Modern dietary advice wrongly encourages us to get lots of insoluble fiber from grain products—or worse, isolated supplements that provide absolutely nothing but a highly processed source of insoluble fiber. This fiber folklore originated with Denis Burkitt, a missionary doctor who was, as an article on him in the *Journal of Nutrition* put it, "well known for his numerous slides of human feces"—photographs he took in Africa during his epidemiological data-finding missions. In 1957 he discovered—or so he thought—that the cause of Western disease was a lack of dietary fiber, specifically from grains. He was the first to make the claim that fiber protected against colon cancer, a claim that has since been debunked. Burkitt felt that the quality and frequency of our stool was a window into the many consequences of our fiber failings. Americans just weren't pooping to his satisfaction.

Here's what Burkitt failed to see: He wasn't observing a low intake of fiber among Americans so much as he was observing a high intake of refined foods, which very likely does play a part in modern Western disease. While refined foods have indeed been stripped of their fiber, that certainly doesn't mean that processed whole-wheat bread is any better for our health than the white stuff. Yet, like Kellogg, Burkitt fixated on fiber, specifically the insoluble kind from grains, and since the time was ripe for the processed-grain industry, Burkitt's agenda was adopted and aided by the very same industries that would have us eat their products. The focus on grain fiber hasn't always been a foregone conclusion. It's a phenomenon that arose right alongside modern myths about fat, cholesterol, and animal foods.

Dietary fiber is composed of indigestible polysaccharides and comes in several forms, the best known being soluble and insoluble fiber. Resistant starch, my "honorary fiber," is less well known. *Indigestible* simply means that it cannot be broken down by our own digestive enzymes. Instead of being digested and absorbed in the small intestine, like starch, sugar, and micronutrients, fiber reaches the large intestine intact.

While most fiber-rich foods contain both soluble and insoluble fiber, the latter often gets the spotlight while the former is forgotten. This is unfortunate, because soluble fiber is well worth remembering—it's just as important as its overexposed counterpart. Soluble fiber attracts water and can expand into a filling, mucilaginous mass that helps keep digestion, especially of sugars, proceeding at an ideal pace, which is a perfect complement to the starch it often comes packaged with in vegetables and fruits: The soluble fiber helps moderate the blood-sugar hit from starch.

Once soluble fiber reaches the large intestine, the veritable poo-poo platter (sorry, couldn't resist) of beneficial bacteria in the colon set about fermenting it and generating anti-inflammatory short-chain fatty acids, which are used as energy by the colonic cells. Resistant starch, found in small amounts in some soluble-fiber-rich foods, is also fermented by the gut bacteria and is an excellent source of butyrate, or butyric acid, the anti-inflammatory short-chain fatty acid you learned about in chapter 2. Because of their ability to feed good gut bacteria, soluble fiber and resistant starch are termed *prebiotics*.

The other kind of fiber—insoluble fiber—is quite different, despite the fact that it's often packaged in the same foods with soluble fiber. Some insoluble fiber is fermentable, and some is not. The most well-known insoluble fiber is cellulose, which is present in the cell walls of plants and is the fiber that both grains and vegetables are touted for. Only minimally fermentable but best known for its indigestibility, cellulose adds bulk but not nutrition and passes right on through the body—and sometimes it causes a little ruckus on the way out.

Most health-care practitioners who encourage us to eat more fiber are talking about the insoluble fiber found in grains, as if grains were the sole source of the stuff. They make this recommendation on the premise that it is "like a broom" in the way it helps "sweep out" the intestines, enabling us to empty our bowels frequently and quickly. What this says to me is that we're all eating such idiotic food that we're constipated enough to think running a broom across our insides to "sweep them out" is a fabulous idea.

We're not supposed to need a butt broom to go number two. That's just a fact.

In recent years, gastroenterologists have begun to catch on to the fact that insoluble fiber from grains is not the only player in the game, especially in cases of digestive distress or gastrointestinal disease, despite their long-standing recommendations to get lots of the stuff when your bowels aren't properly bowel-ing. For those with GI problems, emphasizing grains for insoluble fiber just adds a layer of potential inflammation onto an already-damaged gut.

From a digestive standpoint, it is not insoluble fiber that determines whether we "go." We have a whole team at work in keeping us regular, actually: It is adequate dietary fat, which is digestible; soluble fiber, which is fermentable; *and* insoluble fiber that keep our digestive machinery running smoothly. When it comes to both types of fiber, we just don't need grains with all their other baggage. We can get it all, every last speck we need, soluble and insoluble, fermentable and unfermentable, from fruits and vegetables.

You'll notice that I haven't made much mention of how much fiber we need and how often we need it. That's intentional. While fiber, especially soluble but also insoluble, is a perfectly healthful, natural part of a diet that includes carbohydrate from fruits and vegetables, the amount that feels best can only be determined at an individual level. In other words: Eat fruits and vegetables, both starchy and non-starchy, green, leafy, and otherwise, and pay attention to how you feel. The most important takeaway is that insoluble fiber from grains and supplements is not a cure-all or even a good tool for digestive health. Its emphasis is yet another myth of conventional wisdom.

Fiber is a good thing in natural, appropriate amounts from healthy, unprocessed foods. Whatever fiber we need—insoluble fiber to keep digestion flowing, soluble fiber to keep good bacteria fermenting—we can get from fruits and vegetables. Starchy fruits and vegetables are great sources of soluble fiber, and they also contain insoluble fiber; leafy greens are known for their insoluble fiber, but many are also excellent sources of soluble fiber.

Sing it with me: There is nothing good in grains—including fiber—that we can't get from vegetables and fruits with more nutrition and less baggage.

So if crops like grains, beans, and soy are fighting us at every bite with phytic acid and lectins, and we don't need them for fiber, why have humans been eating grains for tens of thousands of years? Why have beans, as well as corn and rice (both grains), been a part of many healthy cultures' diets for centuries? Doesn't that debunk the whole premise of the Paleo diet?

Not at all, as it turns out. There's a historical and biological context behind everything. It's just a little longer than a sound bite.

After agriculture:
Traditional food, traditional
cultures, traditional preparation

No discussion of the eating habits of our ancestors would be complete without a discussion of our agricultural history and what it truly means to us modern folk.

We generally mark the advent of agriculture—the Agricultural Revolution—at ten thousand to thirty thousand years ago because we have anthropological evidence of grain consumption around that period. But there's a "but," and a big one at that (and you know how much I like big buts): The shift toward agriculture was not quick, and it certainly wasn't based on some delusion about the health properties of grains.

So what drove the transition from hunting to farming, which eventually led to today's agricultural paradigm? A combination of factors, probably on a continuum that flowed from hunting to herding (which kept the food supply close) and cultivating selected plants, all of which led to the ability to stay in one place permanently and produce a survival-ensuring surplus that included both animals and plants. In the slow, self-perpetuating expansion of this way of life, which occurred over thousands of years, the early agriculturalists steadily pushed the wilderness—and their hunter-gatherer past—further out of memory. Communities grew, then cities, then civilizations. Even though herding and crop cultivation required more labor than hunting and gathering, building a reliable, stationary food supply meant a more secure chance at survival based simply on the availability of calories—not nutrients. Short story: Just because they ate it doesn't mean it was good for them.

A common argument about the Agricultural Revolution's negative impact on humanity states that humans developed health problems directly attributable to a crop-based diet. However, the backbreaking work of harvesting crops was undoubtedly involved as well. In large agricultural societies, like that of ancient Egypt, those doing the harvesting developed severe arthritic deformities characteristic of harvest work. Bones from that era show that humans became smaller and weaker and that diseases of nutritional deficiency and infection became more common. In other words, agriculture broke the human body through both hard labor and lesser nutrition, and it would likely do the same today if we hadn't found ways around those issues. Most of us have never grown our own grains or worked our own fields, so we have no idea what it takes to produce the foods we eat; and the grains we do eat are fortified, enriched, and topped off with a Flintstones Kids multivitamin. (Ironic!)

That said, today's grains are vastly different from ancient ones, and ancient agriculturalists didn't suddenly become grain-eating vegetarians sucking down modern wheat. Ancient grains were wild-harvested and unmodified, grown in richer soil without industrial pesticides. Though nutritionally inferior to a hunter-gatherer diet based on animals and forage, they were nowhere near as problematic as today's grains, which are products of industry more than the Earth. Humans didn't simply give up the nutrition they'd long gleaned from animals as agriculture expanded, either, though their animals certainly weren't relegated to factory farms to be fed crop oil industry by-products.

As grains were being cultivated in this new era of agriculture, animals were still kept and used for work and food. Along with the domestication of animals came the consumption of dairy, which likely first occurred around nine thousand years ago. It was quite an ingenious discovery, really: Dairy consumption provided concentrated, calorie-rich, animal-based nutrition that was consistently available, in contrast to having to kill an animal for a one-off shot at its meat.

But keep in mind that this ancient dairy bore absolutely no resemblance to the mass-produced, low-fat, ultra-processed garbage that's a staple in most of our modern-day diets (poured over processed grain, most likely). Today's industrial dairy production practices damage and strip a food that was once nutritious and turn it into an allergenic, industrialized disaster: Homogenization can oxidize and damage dairy fat; skimming removes fat-soluble vitamins A and D; and biologically inappropriate animal feed creates dairy that's fundamentally nutritionally unsound in the first place. Pasteurization actually destroys the beneficial microbes and enzymes in dairy, and it was first adopted not because the unpasteurized stuff was inherently dangerous but because in the early 1800s dairy cows were, for the first time, being kept in "distillery dairies" and fed the by-product of liquor production in what was called the "slop milk industry." Those distillery by-products made cows so sick that they produced equally unhealthy milk, giving all dairy, and nearly nine thousand years of dairy history, a bad name. At its best, dairy is a perfectly nutritious food with a long history in the human diet. At its worst, it's an industrial tragedy.

Here's the point: Food, and the work required to cultivate it, was fundamentally different during the Agricultural Revolution. The wheat was different. The meat was different. The dairy was different. While the anthropology is fascinating and the time line interesting, and it gives some hints as to how we got to where we are today, it's clearly only part of the larger picture. We can't use the advent of agriculture as our only context when it comes to eating similar to—or different from—the humans who lived before it. That'd be a sound bite, and we want a mouthful so big we can't say "chubby bunny."

We can talk agriculture and wheat to the ends of the Earth, but the clues we need aren't buried tens of thousands of years in the past. They're visible in the modern world in nutritional science, which teaches us about the way food affects our bodies, and in the foods traditional cultures eat and how they prepare them. We've talked about nutritional science. Now let's talk about traditional cultures.

The agricultural time line isn't the only time line in human nutrition. There are cultures across the globe that entered the modern era untouched by mass agriculture and processed food—living examples of the health properties of real, nourishing food. Fourteen of these cultures were observed and studied by Weston Price, a dentist who traveled the world in the 1930s, observing and documenting in detail the dietary patterns of healthy and isolated indigenous cultures and tribes. These groups included Swiss and Gaelic cultures, Aboriginal Australians, the Maori of New Zealand, and native Alaskans, all of which are untouched by modern agriculture. He found all of them to be remarkably healthy and free of the diseases of modern civilization, as long as they remained true to the traditional diets their respective cultures had relied on for centuries. When they deviated from tradition, however, and began eating modern, processed foods, health disaster ensued.

Their traditional diets were filled with foods that have always been food, from the Paleolithic era through the Neolithic era through today: foods like meat, fat, and dairy from healthy animals; wild-caught seafood; and plants grown in healthy soil. While each culture ate foods unique to its region, the common ground between them is telling: Their

173

diets provided copious minerals and fat-soluble vitamins, most notably from creature foods, and when they ate the more perilous plants, they prepared them with great care.

They were old-school people living in modern times, relying on collective wisdom and common sense. That, friends, is exactly what living Paleo is all about.

These are the cultures that we can best learn from, that have taught us lessons that are truly applicable to our modern lives. They knew about the problems inherent in certain foods, like grains and beans, long before modern science revealed them, and they developed many ingenious ways to make certain plants safer to eat. They had no other choice. They didn't have an organic grocer on every corner or a supply line to ship in food from thousands of miles away, so they were limited to the food that could be found in their regions. They had to find ways to make potentially problematic food work for them.

For some cultures, that food included wheat and other grains like barley, oats, rye, corn, and rice, as well as beans and other legumes. Though none of these foods resembled the modern, agribusiness-bred, genetically modified, pesticide-resistant, mass-produced, USDA-endorsed junk that we're encouraged to eat today, they still had those pesky compounds—lectins and phytic acid—that made them less digestible and their nutrition less available.

So these cultures developed and passed down ways of breaking down these compounds. They soaked, sprouted, and fermented their problematic plants—often for days and weeks at a time—to break down toxins or trick seeds into germinating, which deactivates phytic acid and allows plants to release their bound-up nutrients. Rice was polished to remove the fibrous bran, where these compounds are found. True sourdough bread, although hard to find today, is fermented, which not only helps break down difficult-to-digest foods but also adds beneficial bacteria to further aid digestion. Latin American cultures' historical means of processing maize, which is still used today, involves a highly alkaline solution that helps remove the antinutrient-rich seed coating and allows minerals and B vitamins—previously inaccessible thanks to phytic acid—to become more bioavailable. Extended soaking and prolonged wet-heat cooking can break down lectins in beans and legumes; without prolonged soaking, most beans are inedible. Fascinatingly, Cate Shanahan notes in her book *Deep Nutrition* that "For the majority of human history, life-giving bread was made not with flour, but with partially germinated seeds." But the critical step of germination is no longer used, and modern bread is made directly from the unsprouted seeds rich in problematic compounds.

These are all fascinating tricks of traditional wisdom, but remember, they were born of necessity. They also don't completely remove the antinutritional properties of those plants. Given our wide range of food choices, we don't have to soak, sprout, or ferment foods of inferior nutrition, nor do we have to make nutritional compromises due to living in isolation as those cultures did.

The bottom line is this: Plants are complicated territory, and, as with fats and meats, it's important to be informed. Humans may have eaten plants since the dawn of time (or, in the case of grains, for a few thousand years; or, in the case of modern grains, for a few decades), but eating smart is about combining the lessons of biology, history, and tradition.

So what to do?

Just eat the good stuff.

When we live on carbage, we're not only working against our energy levels, our sleeping patterns, our blood-sugar regulation, and our moods; we're also working against our digestive systems. That's just the physiology of it. Strangely enough, if we live on "healthy whole grains" and model our diet on the government's recommendations, we're doing the same thing. It's all carbage, and it's all dangerous.

In the immortal words of George Bailey: It's poison, I tell ya. It's poison.

If your food has a label, read it. I always encourage people to do so, but not because I advocate food that requires ingredients labels in the first place. It's more because I like witnessing those "holy crap" moments when the realization hits that we've been tricked into thinking that something in a box with a list smacked on the side is, in some way, food. It's not. It's not food. It. Is. Not. Food.

The only food is the food that has always been food.

Most labels are attached to processed, refined, boxed, or bagged carbage. These products can cause digestive damage and blood-sugar problems, and some grains can even trigger autoimmune disease and other inflammation-related problems. They don't tell ya that on the labels—yet another reason to choose foods that don't need labels at all.

Luckily, you don't need a nutrition label or a rogue, anti-establishment scientist at the cutting edge of nutritional biochemistry to know that vegetables and fruits are whole, unrefined, and pretty dang likely to be good for you. Growing your own, buying organic, or buying from a trusted local grower makes your healthy fruit 'n' veggie choices ironclad.

Choose safe, unprocessed, nutritious, nourishing, and label-less carb-rich foods: whole vegetables and fruits of all kinds. I'm talking about the starchier ones, like roots, squash, tubers, potatoes (yes, potatoes), bananas, and plantains, and the sweet ones, like apples and mangos. I'm also talking about the fibrous ones, like leafy green vegetables and berries. Eat these foods as part of a diet rich in healthy fats and protein so your body gets everything it needs—and less of what it doesn't.

Eat the right amount of carbs for your individual needs, not the amount set forth by a government full of agricultural industry hacks.

But how can we ever know how many carbohydrates we need? Step one: Stop worrying! We all need to get out of our own heads when it comes to carbohydrates. Don't let yourself make this an impossible task of calculating how much of the good stuff is okay and guessing which corner of the Internet is going to give you the perfect read on carbohydrate rules and ratios. Just give yourself some time to figure it out. Don't get lost in the minutiae. All you really need to do is have the patience to observe your body's responses to a variety of real, nutrient-rich food. If it's the good stuff, you've fought 90 percent of the battle already.

From there, you can tweak your diet based on how much carb feels right. An endurance athlete may feel most comfortable with some extra carb-dense foods like sweet potatoes, white potatoes, plantains, and other fruit—or not. A less-active person may feel better with fewer carbs from less-starchy vegetables, like carrots or greens, and lower-sugar fruits like berries—or not. On slow, lazy days, fewer carbs are probably appropriate, unless you feel otherwise. On days you're sprinting after a rogue toddler or saving the world from a zombie invasion, you may want that extra banana. Then again, you may not.

Evaluate how you feel day to day. Do you have steady energy? Are you sleeping well and waking up refreshed? Do you coast into your next meal feeling ready to eat but not starving and cranky? Once you can answer "yes" to those questions, you've found the sweet spot.

The bottom line: Ditch the carbage. Choose real food. Slow down, don't stress, and enjoy.

Chapter 4

nutrients

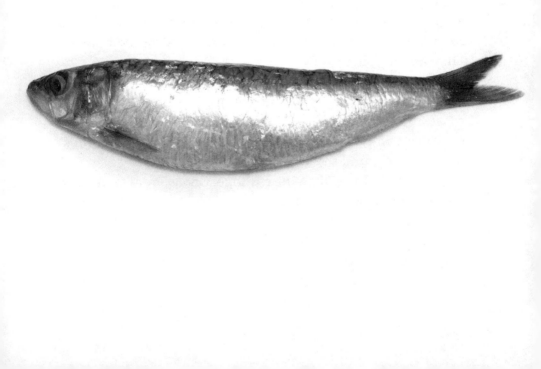

We've talked about all the myths and truths about fat, protein, and carbs. We've talked about what constitutes "real food." But even the most dedicated dogma-bomber can fall victim to deep-seated myths about how our bodies use food and where nutrition truly comes from.

Everything we thought we knew about how nutrients work in our bodies and what we need from our food is wrong—as wrong as soy bacon, margarine, and egg-white omelets.

First, let's talk about the elephant in the room: calories.

On the list of things that matter about our food, calories are dead last.

This is a hard sell, I know. But whether you want to lose weight, gain weight, or simply learn more about what you're putting in your mouth while staying healthy and happy, the last thing that'll get you there is caring about, obsessing over, or counting those calories. It's a waste of energy. Pun intended.

This may sound crazy. Everyone from the fitness fanatics at the local gym to the weight-loss gurus of prime-time television tells us that calorie counting is priority one. We've heard success stories from those who swear by the calorie-counting strategy for losing, gaining, or maintaining weight (although, for this chapter, we'll focus on the most common desire, weight loss). But somehow, it never seems to happen for us. Most of us have tried some form of calorie tracking, with varying levels of temporary success and, of course, epic failure.

Despite all the buzz, the majority of calorie-concerned folks are still storing more than they're burning and rebounding more than they're succeeding, even after their best efforts to restrict, cut back, count calories, and diet. What should that tell us?

I'll tell ya what that should tell us: that restricting, cutting back, counting calories, and dieting. Do. Not. Work. And that's not because the people trying are willpower-less, or unlucky, or destined to be overweight and unhappy. They don't work because they absolutely cannot, never have, and never will accord with our biochemistry. Not in the real world.

Sure, when folks are stuck on a ranch with screaming trainers and personal chefs, these strategies work—for a time. But real-life choices are driven not by the rules of food jail but by individual biochemistry. Against a backdrop of restriction and the metabolic disaster that ensues, there's not a lot of hope for long-term success.

Behind the temporary successes, the ultimate failures, and the caloric folklore is a story that goes far beyond calories. The beast-sized myth that calories matter is in dire need of a shakedown, and it starts with talking about the way things *actually* work. The only way to eat this elephant is one bite at a time, so let's get chewin'.

Calories, energy, and food

When we talk about calories, we're actually talking about the energy we get from the food we eat. Kind of.

See, one food calorie (which is actually a kilocalorie) represents the amount of energy needed to heat one kilogram of water by one degree Celsius.

So what does that tell us about how food acts in our bodies?

In truth, not much, and that's why counting calories—how many go in and how many are being burned—simply doesn't work in the long term. Yet we keep holding on to the calories-in, calories-out model as if somehow, one day, we'll get our bodies to fall in line with it.

We've been taught to think about the food we eat and how it affects our weight and our health solely in terms of calories, despite the fact that the food-as-calories concept is as dated as tapered jeans. It took root nearly 120 years ago, around 1894, and we continue to act as if that's the whole dang story—even though the following century of scientific advancement saw the discovery of several key metabolism-regulating hormones that matter far more than calories. (We'll get to that.)

Why does the calorie count hang around this way, then, if it's not the most important measure of how our bodies handle food? It's hard to say. Partly because it's simple, perhaps, and we're used to it. Partly because the processed-food industry prefers that we think only about calories and never about nutrition. Partly because it's profitable for many diet-food pushers and the weight-loss industry (it would be much harder to assign Weight Watchers points to our hormone levels).

But the way our bodies use food is orders of magnitude more intricate than a simple count of calories eaten and burned, and our metabolism are driven by complex interactions of nutrients, vitamins, minerals, hormones, and things with nerdy acronyms like ATP and BMR. These facts don't change.

BMR, or basal metabolic rate, is an acronym that most of us have probably heard of. I used to spend hours obsessing over it in my quest to change my body. I didn't understand that BMR isn't the approximate measure of how much we need to restrict our calorie intake in order to "get skinny." It's actually just an approximation of the bare minimum amount of energy we need to fuel all the incredible things our bodies do when we aren't physically moving at all.

The millions upon millions of chemical reactions that take place when we're at rest, including those that power a healthy metabolism, require an astounding amount of energy. Running a half-marathon uses less energy than our bodies require for a full day of chemical reactions alone. And for years I was dead-set on shortchanging and underfeeding those chemical reactions so I could look like a Hollywood bobblehead. *What was I thinking?*

Every single thing our bodies do—from lying in bed to running half-marathons to thinking, digesting, moving nutrients across cell membranes, and even turning the pages of a book—requires energy. Food provides the raw materials for energy ("calories in"), and we're told that to change our bodies we have to manipulate both the incoming calories and the amount of energy we expend ("calories out"). And so we wave our pom-poms and cheer for Team Calorie as if it's the metabolic be-all and end-all of the weight game.

But there's more to it than that. In order to lay claim to the energy contained in our food and stored in our bodies, and in order to burn it, certain things have to happen. A bite of broccoli doesn't travel directly to your brain to power an hourlong daydream about Ryan Gosling or Megan Fox. Food, just like body fat, must be metabolized before it means anything to our bottom line. Calories are nothing but an approximation of *potential* energy until our metabolism gets crackin'.

When the body breaks down the fat, protein, and carbs in the foods we eat, it converts them into adenosine triphosphate (ATP), the units of energy that fuel our cells. The creation of ATP is the process of generating energy from food. This process is called *cellular respiration*. This is metabolism at the most fundamental level: It's cellular metabolism, and ATP is what our bodies take to the energy bank. It supplies the energy for everything our cells do, from coordinating the movement of our muscles to powering our organs. ATP, not calories, is our true "cellular money," and it's where energy actually comes from. Calories? That's just a number on the nutrition label.

ATP is created on demand, based on the needs of the moment. We don't store ATP in our bodies in any appreciable amount—just enough for a few seconds of activity—but we do store the raw materials for making it, lickety-split, when we need it. We get these raw materials from the food we eat and store them in our muscles, liver, and—yes—body fat.

Now we're getting somewhere.

So how do we access body fat to use it for ATP?

As we've discussed, the way our bodies create and use energy is far more complex than we've been told. It should come as no surprise, then, that storing fat, burning fat, losing weight, and maintaining true health at any given moment is an equally elaborate prospect.

It's the hormones, honey

We're going to talk about body fat right now. But we're not going to talk about getting skinny, getting lean, getting ripped, getting a dancer's body, getting a CrossFit body, getting an apple bottom, bulking, mass-gaining, getting shredded, or achieving any body type that's not your body's own natural manifestation of health. If you're looking to push your body to be something it's not naturally designed to be, it's a cold, hard fact that you may sacrifice your long-term health in the process. I can't help you do that. Doesn't feel right.

Why? Because I want you to be healthy first and foremost, before you try to do anything else. It's the best possible foundation you can give yourself for anything and everything you want to be, do, and achieve. Put *that* on a unicorn poster.

Some of us are naturally inclined to be thin and lean in our greatest state of health. Some of us are naturally inclined toward bulk or big muscles. Some of us are brick houses with apple bottoms. Some of us are naturally curvy and full-bodied. We are healthiest when we feel good, when we're well nourished, when our bodies are balanced rather than hoarding or wasting, and when we shut off that judge-y internal monologue that says, *I can only read books about food that tell me how to look like Sparkles McCelebrity.* You'll look better as a healthy you than you would as an imitation *them* anyway.

All that said, it's still critical to dismantle the rest of the calorie mythology so that if you need to lose or gain weight, get healthy, or just be wicked smart, you've got the facts.

Our body fat level—how much we store and how much we're able to recruit to burn—is a function of our metabolism. This is true for everyone from rail-thin beanpoles to the morbidly obese and everyone in between. And our ability to metabolize stored body fat in that ATP-generating cellular furnace is not a calories-in, calories-out operation. It's a product of our hormones.

I repeat: It's not about calories. It's about hormones.

Hormones have their say before, during, and after meals. Every food you eat and every calorie that comes along for the ride is at the mercy of your hormones.

Sometimes, our bodies become adapted to a weight or a state that just doesn't feel right. However we got there, our bodies want, more than anything, to maintain the balance they've achieved. That's why we can't always get our bodies to do what we want them to do: When we ask them—through diet, exercise, or a combination of the two—to leave the state to which they've adjusted, they'll hang on to the status quo at almost any cost. They'll throw fits in the form of depressed metabolism, fatigue, or wild hunger pangs, which drive us to keep fat in storage and keep more food coming in. These diet nightmares are not consequences of a lack of willpower. They're consequences of the hard work our hormones are doing to keep our bodies where they've adapted to be.

And this isn't because hormones are schoolyard bullies that want to make us miserable for no good reason. Our bodies are programmed to use hormones to store raw materials and maintain our weight whenever possible for the sake of survival because, for millions of years of human evolution, food was not guaranteed as it is for most of us today. In this era of constantly flowing food, however, these hormones are operating in overdrive to make a now-obsolete survival scenario possible.

This makes harnessing our hormone function all the more important, because our environment isn't gonna do it for us.

The hormonal control of our metabolism involves thyroid function, cortisol, and a range of other organs, tissues, and hormones, but the most important orchestrators to understand are the hormones insulin and leptin. Insulin and leptin are responsible, respectively, for storing energy in our fat cells and then maintaining those stores, and they can't be manipulated by counting calories. In fact, conventional diet behavior—avoiding dietary fat and counting calories—works against hormonal harmony in every way. A low-fat diet rich in carbohydrates is insulin's fat-storage dream, and a low-calorie diet sends leptin on a mission to get you eating again.

Insulin: The hoarder

Insulin, which is produced by the pancreas (yet another process that requires ATP), is responsible for transporting glucose—which is derived from carbohydrates—from our blood to our cells, where it is stored. Our liver cells get their fill of glucose first, followed by our muscle cells. Then the remaining glucose is converted to triglycerides and stored in our fat cells for the next famine—or at least our bodies *think* it's being stored for the next famine. But that famine never happens, and the food keeps coming.

So, thanks to insulin, whatever carbohydrate we don't burn is stored as fat. That doesn't make carbs bad, of course, but it does explain why too many carbs too often—a frequent scenario brought on by the low-fat, high-carb diet of conventional wisdom, which is heavy in too many insulin-spiking, nutrient-stealing, processed carbohydrates and low in healthy fats, protein, and slow-digesting starches—turns us into unwitting fat hoarders.

Speaking of insulin, there's a reason lower-carb diets have been shown to be more effective for weight loss than low-fat, high-carb ones: Restricting carbohydrates lends us a greater degree of hormonal control in our quest to conquer fat stores. Basically, they tell insulin to take a chill lozenge, allowing us to access stored body fat.

To a point, having that "little something extra" just means that your body is prepared for anything that demands extra energy, from famine, to bouts of intense exercise like flash-mob marathons, to growing a tiny person in your uterus. But well beyond that *little something* is that *lot of something,* and once we cross the threshold from metabolically aligned and well nourished to overburdened by too many junk carbohydrates and too little true nutrition, we go from healthy and prepared to hormonally handicapped.

Excessive storage of body fat begins with the never-ending demand we place on insulin production thanks to a diet based on more carbohydrates than we are able to burn. Our individual storage tanks fill well beyond the body's short- and long-term energy needs, and this cycle continues as long as we keep eating a steady stream of processed carbohydrates. At the same time, the constant rise and fall of blood sugar drives us to eat more than we normally would—which has nothing to do with calories and everything to do with hormonal control. The job of a hormone is to communicate, and insulin is saying, *Store, store, store.*

When we eat more carbs than our bodies can handle and the excess overwhelms our individual tolerance for too long, the consequences reach far beyond fat storage. The constant barrage of insulin on our cells can become like white noise. Our cells tune it out, and yet another metabolic horror takes root: insulin resistance, also known as metabolic syndrome, wherein the cells no longer respond to the message of insulin, ceasing to allow glucose into the cells. This leaves blood glucose constantly high—a condition that is inflammatory, a precursor to type 2 diabetes, and a risk factor for heart disease.

And while all this is happening, the body is working to maintain itself under these conditions, striving to adjust to its circumstances while hanging on to what it's been given. This makes it much more difficult to make changes through conventional caloric restriction, willpower, or dieting, which work against what the body is programmed to do.

Says who? Says leptin.

Leptin: The bond company stooge

If insulin is the energy hoarder, leptin is the body's bond company stooge: on-site 24/7 to ensure that the body doesn't try any funny business. Leptin has the final word on all things metabolism-related.

Leptin is a hormone produced by fat cells whose purpose is to protect body fat stores to increase our chances of survival. Where insulin is a storage hormone, leptin is a "Nobody gets out of this fat cell unless I say so" hormone. When we diet, restrict calories, or do anything jarring or drastic in an attempt to drop fat, it's leptin that drops instead, and when leptin levels plummet, several fat-loss fail-safes are activated: Metabolic rate drops, ravenous hunger sets in, and fatigue drives us to conserve energy. In short, leptin drives the dreaded rebound.

Ever had an overwhelming desire to break your diet three days in, skip spin class, and sit on the couch with a box of Krispy Kremes? Yeah. That was leptin's idea.

Leptin can be extremely bossy with other hormones as well. When it's out of balance, leptin can manipulate thyroid function and sex hormones. Add falling asleep mid-interlude to the doughnuts and couch-surfing, and you've got the full angry leptin experience.

I'm mostly joking, of course, but here's the point: Sometimes we think there's something wrong with our commitment or our willpower to cut calories when in fact it's just our hormones telling us that they won't give up without a fight. Once we've consumed and conserved sufficient energy to bring fat stores back to their original state, leptin returns to normal and appetite levels off—and all the while, we may not have realized that leptin was in control.

Sound like doom-and-gloom? It's not. It's just another survival mechanism, and it doesn't take kindly to threats. But it does explain why calorie-counting and dieting don't work—biology trumps force of will.

While our appetites go back to normal once leptin is back at normal levels, if we're fueled by the wrong foods—like nutrient-poor, insulin-spiking ones—we never really respond appropriately to that drop in appetite. And if we keep indulging, the constant barrage of insulin can cause an overproduction of leptin, making the brain become resistant to leptin's signals. Since leptin is what gives us a feeling of satiety when we're full, our hunger can become excessive and relentless, just as it can when we restrict food. Fatigue can become debilitating. Weight loss becomes impossible and weight gain inevitable.

It's all about the hormones. Hormones, not lack of willpower, drive hunger and overeating in response to dieting and food restriction. Hormones make us move less—even when we don't realize it—to conserve energy. Hormones drive fat storage and fat burning. Hormones don't play fair, because they operate on the individual level: They can make an overweight person gain weight on a restricted-calorie diet while an underweight person struggles to add pounds no matter how much she eats. Hormones downgrade our metabolic rate when we're restricting calories or stressing our bodies with too little nutrition, and hormones unleash the metabolic burn beast when we nourish our bodies right. (Yeah. I said "metabolic burn beast.")

The good news: If we're well nourished and not antagonizing our bodies with too many processed carbs and an incessant influx of insulin, and if we're not constantly calling on leptin to respond to periods of extreme dieting or deprivation or, alternatively, overindulgence in nutrient-poor food, our hormones are much more likely to throw us a bone and unleash that beast. Insulin can be controlled, and leptin does allow us to burn fat—just not by restricting nourishment.

The path to hormonal balance is also the path to true health: Don't restrict nourishment. Forget about calories. Eat real food.

Processed food, conventional wisdom, and calorie restriction wage war on health and hormonal balance. Crap food simply doesn't stimulate satiety, and it overstimulates fat storage and appetite while leaving us strapped for nutrition and hankering for more, more, more. The result: We eat more than we need while becoming less healthy.

But when we eat real food, we give our bodies what they need to work properly, create energy efficiently, stay full and satisfied, and work their way back to hormonal happiness. Real food fills us up physically: Whole vegetables, fruits, and animal protein are naturally rich in water, and whole vegetables and fruits have the perfect amount of fiber. These foods all digest at a steady pace, keeping us satisfied longer. Real food also satisfies us hormonally: Animal protein and healthy, unprocessed fats provide raw materials that are converted into the hormones that help regulate appetite. Fat, unlike carbohydrate, does not stimulate insulin release. These are real food's natural defenses against overeating and undernourishing.

But, most important, real food supplies micronutrients—vitamins and minerals—that are critical for healthy metabolism. B vitamins are needed for the release of cellular energy and the generation of ATP. Minerals like calcium, magnesium, iron, and zinc are essential for metabolic jobs like moving fats across cell membranes, delivering nutrition from the digestive system into the bloodstream, powering muscle contraction and release, transporting oxygen, and stabilizing cells. Seeking foods rich in nutrients means getting more from our metabolism, whatever the calorie count.

And it's not just our metabolism that benefits from the nourishment in real food. Vitamins and minerals are also our path to overall wellness, healing, and a beautifully healthy body.

Nutrients, not calories

If you leave this literary masterpiece with just one delicious tidbit, let it be this one: The calories in natural, unprocessed, real foods are more than just calories. They're full of more magic than a Disney Princess convention. They come with nutrients that make us healthier, stronger, happier, and more beautiful. They keep us satisfied in more ways than one—a good hunk of butter doesn't just satisfy the appetite, it also satisfies the soul. Cate Shanahan has said, "When a chef talks about flavor, he's also talking about nutrients," and that's true. There isn't a half-decent chef on this planet who will use margarine instead of butter, Crisco instead of lard, or canned broth instead of homemade stock. Customers would leave absolutely unsatisfied—because you can't fake the satisfaction that comes from having eaten food that nourishes.

Okay, so that's more of a tid-bunch. But the real foods I've spent thousands of words blabbing about are pretty major when it comes to nutrition—and, for that reason, they have the power to change your life. Counting calories simply can't do that.

Counting calories doesn't work for your body, mind, or soul. It can't keep the Biggest Losers from becoming the Biggest Regainers. Counting calories can't help your body make hormones that regulate appetite and metabolism. It can't help your body make the neurotransmitters that make you happy or help you wake up feeling refreshed. Counting calories can't help you establish a deeper connection to your own instincts about food, it can't help you know when you're full, and it can't help you stop obsessing.

The diet industry wants us to think about counting calories rather than establishing a baseline of health by nourishing our bodies. They act as if our problems are the result of too many calories when most of us are actually suffering from a nourishment deficiency. A box of industrial crap that promises a low-calorie path to health or weight loss (and most diet systems and prepackaged meals fit that bill) provides nothing but a carnival show—all smoke and mirrors. This is the business of sales, not the business of health, and it leaves us the same or worse off than it found us.

This whole circus does nothing to solve all the issues that we tend to forget can stem directly from nutrient deficiency: fatigue, depression, poor digestion, and weight gain, among others. Funny thought from the girl who used to live on 100-calorie packs: Ever wonder why they don't call it a 100-nutrient pack?

The problem is, we don't think about food in terms of nourishment. We think of food as a calorie-laden nemesis, and we think of appetite as something we must control with the only tool we have: willpower. Well, I no longer believe in willpower. I believe in a body that's nourished enough to know what it needs and when. It's possible. But the diet and processed-food industries would rather you didn't know that. The diet industry, in particular, wants you to think of food in terms of weight loss first, and I don't believe in that, either. If your only goal is to lose weight and you don't care about nourishing your body with good nutrition, I'm surprised you made it this far. Maybe you're actually looking for something more.

Eating and appreciating real food allows your instincts to kick in. If you silence the inner calorie-crazy, your body will begin to tell you when it's gotten the nutrition it desperately needs. You'll notice the changes.

Calories are simply not created equal. A calorie's worth of real food does more for your health, your body, and your goals than a calorie's worth of conventional junk. Think of it this way: A pound of pennies weighs the same as a pound of quarters, but how much more is the pound of quarters worth?

I despise math but I love money, so I can tell you this: A pound of pennies is worth a pittance, just $1.81. A pound of quarters is worth a full twenty bucks. I want the pound with the most money. (I can buy better food with it.)

So let's ditch the calorie-counting myth. I'm over the obsessing. The rest of this chapter is dedicated to what actually matters. I don't care about counting calories. I care about banking nourishment.

Nutrients: Bank them, and bank on them

Our entire sensibility surrounding food is one of restriction, and that's been the theme for at least fifty years: Restrict calories. Restrict fat. Restrict cholesterol. Restrict animal products. Don't eat too much of whatever processed food you replace them with. And don't worry about the nutrients that you're restricting in the process.

But when we restrict food—in particular, robust, nutrient-dense food—we restrict nutrition. Talk about breaking the bank. This way of eating makes meager nutrient deposits and major withdrawals, gradually depleting our nutrients and blunting our efforts to feel our best. What we need is not fewer calories or less of the foods our ancestors ate. What we need is less crap food, less diet dogma, and unlimited deposits of good nutrition. And maybe a few more bank analogies.

Nutrients protect us from chronic disease, bolster our immunity, protect our fertility, balance hormones and hunger, build healthy skin and teeth, cushion our joints, and keep anti-inflammatory processes in balance. When we're nutrient-depleted, our bodies simply don't run as they should. We can see a whole culture of depletion around us: chronic disease, infertility, skin disorders, mouths full of dental work, obesity, and joint problems. All this because our food supply and our dietary dogma have failed us. They've led us to become deficient not just in the right fats, protein, and carbs, but also in precious nutrients.

Need specifics? The above conditions are impacted by vitamins A, D, E, and K_2; B vitamins; and minerals like zinc, iron, calcium, and magnesium, many of which I'll talk about as the chapter goes on. They're all involved. And the beautiful part is that all these nutrients are found in real food, together, in the right amounts, just waiting to make us healthier.

Notice that I said *real food*. Unfortunately, the habitual popping of vitamin pills can't bring us back from the brink.

Part of the reason supplements aren't a substitute for good nutrition is that they simply can't replicate the magic of real food. Nutrients occur together in nature for a reason. For example, foods rich in calcium, such as sardines and raw milk, are also naturally rich in vitamin D, which helps the body utilize calcium. This synergy can't be replicated in a lab-created pill. To make the story even more grim, many multivitamins are filled with partial, fractionated, or synthetic substitutes for the nutrients they're meant to replace.

I don't say this to make life difficult. Exactly the opposite: I'm trying to take some of the trepidation out of healthy living. I'm trying to give back the thousands of hours most of us have spent in the supplement aisle sleuthing vitamins and the hundreds of dollars we've spent trying to get all the nutrition we need from a shopping cart full of pills.

The nutrition we need is generally found all in one place—not in a bottle or a capsule, and not even in vegetables and fruits alone, but in properly raised animal foods.

Sounds carnivorous, I know, but this book is certainly not a meat-only manifesto. I adore vegetables, especially when they're drenched in butter or served with a grass-fed steak (wink), and I'm known to go fruit-crazy from time to time. But we can't get bankable nutrition from plants alone. We actually need the fat-soluble vitamins found in animal foods to use the water-soluble vitamins found in plants, so there's truly no way around it: We have to get nutrition from animal sources, and we'd be well served to prioritize quality animal nutrition above all else.

Lose the Bambi baggage

If we let go of our baggage about saturated fats from animals, about fat in general, and about animal protein and we start identifying the foods with the greatest nutritional value as the best foods, the conclusion is clear: My crack team of Paleo foods wins. It wins every single time.

And if I had to pick a captain for Team Paleo, it would be properly raised or wild-hunted animals and wild-caught fish—both, not either/or. Not only do these foods contain healthy fats, but they're also packed with those critical fat-soluble vitamins in their active forms. The nutrients found in animal foods are so important that our bodies are able to store them for emergencies, as in the case of B_{12}, and sometimes, under the right circumstances, even create them from the raw materials found in plants, as in the case of vitamin A and the end-usable form of omega-3. The key phrases, however, are *for emergencies* and *under the right circumstances.* Our ability to make and store these nutrients is a physiological redundancy that ensures a temporary supply should we be cut off from the ideal sources. Ya know, just in case the crap hits the fan. Famine. Zombie invasions. Veganism. (I kid.)

Technically, only small quantities of vitamins are needed for normal physiological function, but what this really means is that small amounts are needed to prevent *abnormal* physiological function. A bit of vitamin C may cure scurvy and a smidge of vitamin A may cure night blindness, but this is hardly a recipe for optimal health. Diseases of clinical deficiency like scurvy and night blindness may be rare in the developed world today, but evidence of subclinical deficiency is all around us, and has been for quite some time.

A prime example: Beginning in the early 1900s, grains replaced animal foods as the primary food source in the American diet. In many cases, animal foods became a luxury rather than a staple. As grain-based foods and flours became the main source of calories (and to an even greater extent in more recent history, as highly processed grains and sugar became an ever-larger part of the average diet), the consequences of certain sneaky deficiencies—especially deficiencies in animal-native nutrients like vitamins A, D, and K_2—became more common. These deficiencies are revealed by something we now consider normal: dental problems.

Ever had braces? Wisdom teeth out? Cavities, spacers, or palate expanders? If so, this discussion applies to you. One of the most glaring, and most often forgotten, indications of the so-common-it's-considered-normal nutrient deficiencies in our culture is the imperfect formation of the bones of the face and jaw and consequently misaligned teeth. Vitamins A, D, and K_2 play direct, complementary roles in the formation of our skeletal structures, including our jaw and facial structures, which are designed to be robust and wide and accommodate rows of straight, strong teeth. The consequences of deficiency can take root even before we're born: The first trimester of pregnancy is a critical time for the formation of the jaw and facial structure, and maternal nutrient deficiencies may play a role in the imperfect development of a baby's jaw and palate.

In his 1939 book *Nutrition and Physical Degeneration,* Weston Price observed that indigenous cultures that maintained diets rich in animal-derived, fat-soluble vitamins and minerals, especially during pregnancy, had well-structured faces and jaws with room for every tooth, perfectly aligned, and minimal, if any tooth decay. Neurobiologist and fat researcher Stephan Guyenet remarks that our modern dental issues are "part of a developmental syndrome that predominantly afflicts industrially living cultures." He believes, as I do, that we're meant to have straight teeth, strong dentition, plenty of room for all our teeth, and a well-aligned bite. Yet I had braces, spacers, cavities, and wisdom teeth extractions; my bite is still imperfect; and I grew up in the era of replacing animal fats with vegetable oils, replacing animal products with plants, and following the grain-heavy food pyramid. What about you?

When we look at our modern food supply, it's not difficult to trace the origins of rampant nutrient deficiencies. In turning away from animal foods and opting instead for nutrient-poor grains and crop oils, we've removed natural sources of vitamins A, D, and K_2. Even those who still eat animal products but don't source them from properly raised animals may suffer the same consequences: When animals are raised indoors or on inappropriate feed, their tissues can't concentrate the nutrition that comes from grazing on grass (which ultimately generates vitamins A and K_2) in the afternoon sun (which ultimately generates vitamin D).

There's some awareness of the importance of vitamins A and D in the standard American food paradigm, and we see it in the conventional dairy industry. Unfortunately, this awareness hasn't led to a true improvement in their product. This industry's practices strip milk of its nutritional value not just by keeping dairy cows in pens and giving them inappropriate feed but also through pasteurization, which destroys the usability of natural vitamin D, and skimming, which removes the fat and, with it, any naturally occurring vitamin A. For this reason, the conventional dairy industry "enriches" or "fortifies" their product with often-synthetic vitamins—that's what "vitamin D milk" actually is. The government and most nutrition professionals recommend fortified milk because they know that without fortification, they'd be recommending a product totally devoid of nutrition.

When you see a nutrient like vitamin D on an ingredients list, it's not because the nutrient was present naturally. It's because it was added after the fact, because *we need it and it's not there.* This goes for foods like conventional milk, bread, boxed cereal, and baby food, such as rice cereal, which is far inferior to traditional animal-based nutrition and must be fortified with everything from B vitamins to minerals to make it even marginally nutritious for babies. (If you want baby to get B vitamins, might I suggest you consider some nice beef or bison? Yes, I'm being serious.)

With that in mind, let's continue our myth-smashing journey, beginning with one of the most pervasive nutrition myths on the planet. The nutrients that matter can't make their impact felt unless they're natural, unprocessed, and in forms we can best absorb and use, and once again, animal products are the belle of this ball.

Myth: The nutrients found in animals can also be found in plants

You may have heard a rumor that we don't need to eat animals because we can get the exact same nutrients from plants. Many plant-based dieters and nutrition enthusiasts believe this. Many high-level nutrition professionals and institutions have said it. At one time, I told people the same thing. We were all wrong.

There are, of course, healthy people who eat no animal products at all. Good for them. Ten, twenty, or thirty years down the road, that healthy story may change. There's no statute of limitations on nutrient deficiency—we don't eventually become immune to long-term consequences. But even if we did, what your neighbor does is of no concern to you (unless, of course, your neighbor is force-feeding you canola oil). Eyes on your own plate: What matters is how *you* feel and what *your* instincts tell you is right for you.

We can get many lovely micronutrients from plants, but they are not the same micronutrients we get from eating the flesh of other creatures.

Yes, that sounds intense. But that's the hard fact, and it's part of this biological rock opera called *Life on Earth*. Creatures like animals and fish have a natural ability that serves us *Homo sapiens* well: They convert and concentrate the nutrients in plants, transforming them into the nutrients we need most.

And thank goodness for that, because nutrients don't just appear in our food out of nowhere. Nutrient-rich plants start with the foundation of nutrient-rich soil, because plants take up and concentrate those nutrients. Bugs and animals with appropriately equipped digestive systems eat the plants and convert and concentrate those nutrients further. The same happens in the marine world, where nutrients from algae are concentrated and passed along through small aquatic organisms and fish. We humans eat those animals and fish, the chain continues, and we're gifted with nutrition we can use.

Ruminant animals, such as cows and deer, turn grass and plants composed of cellulose—a form of insoluble fiber that humans cannot digest and that tastes like lawn clippings— into nutritious meat packed with vitamin A, vitamin K_2, protein, zinc, and iron. Algae, which smells like soggy feet, sends omega-3 up the marine food chain to be concentrated in fish that are rich in other nutrients as well, including taurine, coenzyme Q10 (CoQ10), and selenium. These living beings convert nutrients into a form that not only tastes really good but that we can digest and use better than any other. In short, they make more usable nutrients out of less usable ones and package everything in added goodies to top it off.

This is the food chain we learned about in grade school, and it doesn't just exist for our entertainment. It has a purpose. Creatures convert and concentrate nutrients so that bigger creatures, including humans, can make use of them. The food chain isn't just a cutesy little quirk of nature; it's built into our biology. We can either become responsible, respectful stewards of that reality or we can live in denial, punishing our bodies for the way they're meant to work.

The nutrients we get from plants are wonderful, colorful, and healthy, but they are different from the ones we get from creatures. I love my veggies, but they cannot provide the fat-soluble vitamins found in animal foods, which our bodies need to make optimal use of other nutrients, including those from plants. Even special, super-organic, happy-hippie, kale-tastic plants cannot provide us with the fat-soluble vitamins A, D, and K_2. They just can't. So it's imperative to prioritize those quality creature foods.

The sole fat-soluble vitamin found in plant form is vitamin E, which is abundant in red palm oil, nuts, and seeds. It's there for a reason: Vitamin E is an antioxidant that helps protect fragile, easily oxidized polyunsaturated fat, which is found in those very same nuts and seeds. It's no surprise, then, that the more polyunsaturated fat we eat, the more vitamin E we need; and the more polyunsaturated fat in natural food, the more vitamin E is present. See how smart Mother Nature is? This is just one example of the phenomenal synergy of real food.

I've already talked about the myths and truths surrounding the macronutrients fat, protein, and carbohydrate, and I've covered each as it relates to our health. I've talked about the calorie myth and why nutrients are what really matters, and I've talked about the fact that nutrients should come from real food, not fortified foods or supplements, and that animals are the best source for us. I haven't yet talked in depth about a few of my favorite individual micronutrients, however, and this is a critical piece of the puzzle. Though these nutrients are the key to good health and general super-powers, some of them have gotten a not-so-good name. I aim to fix that, for the health of our bodies and our nutrient bank accounts.

And so we continue our myth-busting tour.

Let's talk about my favorite nutrients, the myths surrounding them, and where to find them. While we're at it, let's talk about some falsely demonized nutrients that many of us have gone without because our health professionals simply don't realize how important they are. While these are by no means the only nutrients that matter, they're the ones that most need a little extra PR. Finally, let's talk about truly getting back to the foods our ancestors ate. (That last part will be for badasses only. You'll see.)

Nutrients we need:
A is for *animals only*

....

We're smack in the middle of an era of vitamin A confusion, and it's not because its benefits are unclear. The importance of true vitamin A is well understood in the scientific community—it's critical for immune function, skin health, fetal development, the body's ability to use minerals, lung health, eye health, bone growth, and cancer prevention— yet trusted authorities from the Mayo Clinic to the Harvard School of Public Health juxtapose the exultation of its benefits with half-assed cautionary statements about vitamin A's potential toxicity. The University of Maryland Medical Center website states, after multiple paragraphs touting the importance of vitamin A, that "While vitamin A is essential for good health, it can be toxic in high doses" and that eating fruits and vegetables rich in beta-carotene, a vitamin A precursor, rather than animal foods rich in true vitamin A is an alternative by which you can increase your body's vitamin A levels.

Here's what they're actually saying, if I interpret what I read correctly: "Vitamin A is critical. It is also toxic. It is abundant in animal products, but we should get it from plants. Plants contain beta-carotene, which is different from vitamin A. Beta-carotene is also the same as vitamin A. I dunno, what do you want from me? Is it time for my lunch break yet?"

For obnoxious why-weasels like me, this is confusing and contradictory and stinks of *nobody's bothered to look into this lately*. The current approach to vitamin A in the School of Conventional Wisdom is equivalent to a dismissive shrug. For some reason, educational outlets keep regurgitating the same oppositional phrases, leaving people like me to play WTF Watchdog.

The widespread myth that vitamin A occurs in plants is as false as the eyelashes at the Oscars. A vitamin A precursor called *beta-carotene* is found in brightly colored vegetables like peppers and carrots, but this is absolutely not true vitamin A.

There is no accounting for the belief that vitamin A occurs in plants, except for one tiny little detail: The FDA has allowed beta-carotene to be labeled as vitamin A. Those jokers.

As if this nutritional swindle isn't dumbfounding enough, there's another layer to the dirty dealing. The beta-carotene in many vitamin supplements and fortified foods, which we'd expect to be taken from the same vegetables in which natural beta-carotene is found, are often synthetic, derived not from plants but from petrochemicals. The labels on fortified foods and supplements won't tell you which is which, perhaps because the lab-created nutrients are associated with an increased risk of cancer. (Although how awesome would it be to see the phrase *This shit fake* on a label? I'd buy that just on principle.)

Beta-carotene is termed a *vitamin A precursor* because it can, in some circumstances, through a series of chemical conversions within the human body, be converted into true vitamin A. This was apparently good enough for the FDA to consider them equal; unfortunately, it's not good enough for our bodies. Until the conversion happens, they are entirely different nutrients.

Worse, the body's beta-carotene conversion ratio is poor, and thyroid issues, stress, and a nutrient-poor diet (which is, let's be honest, the Standard American Diet) can all interfere with this conversion. At best, it takes as many as six units of beta-carotene to create one unit of vitamin A.

Imagine that someone gives you six adorable puppies and then says you can only keep one. See? It's sad.

Beta-carotene from plants is converted with great efficiency, however, by the properly raised, wild-hunted, or wild-caught creatures we eat. True vitamin A accumulates in these creatures' tissues, providing a concentrated source for us when we eat them.

The body's beta-carotene-to-vitamin-A conversion that plants-only eaters rely on is meant for emergencies only. It's a physiological redundancy we're fortunate to have and even more fortunate *not* to have to use. Beta-carotene is certainly a lovely plant nutrient, but it's not to be relied on as a source of true vitamin A. The only sources of true vitamin A are creature foods, such as egg yolks, full-fat unprocessed dairy, shellfish, liver, and cod liver oil. (Grow a pair. It's good for you.) Unfortunately, these are the foods many folks won't touch with a ten-foot carrot.

The next component of the vitamin A myth is the belief that true vitamin A from animals can be toxic, despite its extraordinary importance to the human body.

But isn't vitamin A toxic?

A word of caution: Vitamin A derivatives, like those used in skin medications like Accutane and topical retinoids, can cause birth defects and are classified accordingly. But remember, these are entirely different, lab-synthesized forms of vitamin A and are not the same as natural, true vitamin A from animals.

We can trace the vitamin A toxicity myth to a few events and misconceptions brought to light by the investigative work of the Weston A. Price Foundation. In 1995, a study (whose results, incidentally, have never been replicated) claimed that women consuming higher amounts of vitamin A were at high risk for having children with certain birth defects. Though the study had glaring flaws, and though vitamin A–rich foods had long been recommended for pregnant women due to their immense importance to fetal development, the study was picked up by the media, which reported that vitamin A is linked to brain defects in babies. Cue national hysteria.

What really happened in this study? When we take a look behind the curtain, it becomes clear that things aren't what they seem. In brief, the study identified a few trends relating higher vitamin A intake with an increased incidence of birth defects—just a few weak correlations—but alongside these weak correlations were indications of a relationship between vitamin A *deficiency* and birth defects. None of this means much, however, as no effort was made to differentiate between naturally occurring vitamin A from animal foods and the synthetic vitamin A used in supplements and as an additive in refined foods. There was also no accounting for the nutrients that, in nature, often come along with vitamin A, such as zinc and vitamin D, and how those nutrients might affect how vitamin A functions in the body. And all the results have to be taken with a grain of salt because the study relied on participants' recollections of their dietary intake, which are notoriously imprecise.

Too often we take conclusions from flawed studies as gospel without asking questions, and it continues to get us into trouble.

Other suggestions of vitamin A toxicity, including the negative impact of high doses of vitamin A on bone structure, are drawn from multiple animal studies wherein rats, dogs, rabbits, pigs, and chickens were given incredibly high doses of isolated vitamin A—up to thousands of times their biological requirement—which did, indeed, induce toxicity and bone fractures.

In a laboratory, when vitamin A is given in isolation and in excess, we can expect to get isolated, excessive results. We've got to wrap our heads around the fact that laboratory experiments involving one nutrient in isolation aren't representative of the way a nutrient acts in its natural habitat.

If we look at real-world human studies regarding vitamin A and bone health, we find that bone-degrading vitamin A toxicity actually occurs only in the absence of adequate vitamin D, and that when the two nutrients are balanced, they work together to maintain bone structure and strength by governing the critical cycles of building and rebuilding. Luckily, in nature—not in a laboratory and not in a box, bag, or capsule—no nutrient exists in isolation. Vitamin A and vitamin D often occur together in food, as in egg yolks, raw milk, and cod liver oil.

The fact that vitamins A and D frequently occur together in nature is telling. We do need both, not one in isolation, and thankfully the natural world is set up that way. However, that is not to say vitamin A toxicity does not exist. It is possible, if one were eating excessive amounts of extremely vitamin A–rich foods without complementary vitamin D for long periods of time, to induce vitamin A toxicity; this would likely involve extreme dosing of heat-processed cod liver oil (which is low in vitamin D) or extreme amounts of liver, which is extremely rich in vitamin A, in a vitamin D–deficient diet. It is possible, though unlikely, to experience toxicity through a diet based on whole foods rich in all the fat-soluble vitamins. A very good thing, since they're so critical to health.

This gives us critical insight into the incredible, undeniable importance of nutrient synergy. Vitamin A has other accessory nutrients that often occur in the very same foods, and as nature's brilliance would have it, they all work together. Zinc, iron, and vitamin K_2 all interact with vitamin A to keep skin beautiful, eyes sharp, and the immune system strong. They keep lungs healthy. They nourish developing babies. They fight cancer and keep our antioxidant defenses high. Fun fact: Vitamin A is a potent antioxidant, just like cholesterol, which is also found only in animal products. Although we often think that plants are the only source of antioxidant power, animal products actually contain even more.

Luckily, a nutrient-dense diet based on ancestral, Paleo principles provides these nutrients in the natural balance we need.

I can't stress this enough: Nutrient synergy is the reason real, whole foods are good for us and not toxic, as isolated or synthetic nutrients could very well be. It is critical that vitamin A occurs in proportion with other nutrients, including vitamin D, as those nutrients work together.

So we really, really shouldn't forget about our vitamin D.

Nutrients we need:
D is for *don't get deficient*

We can get vitamin D naturally in two ways: through the sun's ultraviolet B (UVB) rays, which stimulate the conversion of cholesterol within our bodies into vitamin D, and in vitamin D–containing foods like egg yolks, lard, cod liver oil, and raw milk. (Plants contain a less biologically active form of vitamin D, which can't provide the same benefits as vitamin D from the sun or creature foods.) Supplements are a third source, often recommended by health professionals as an easy way out of vitamin D deficiency, though it's not an ideal approach: There is evidence that vitamin D supplementation can actually suppress the immune system rather than boost it. For that reason, I'm going to focus on natural sources of vitamin D.

Unlike true vitamin A, which is still a mainstream *nutrient non grata,* vitamin D has been given some well-deserved respect in the last few years, specifically for its importance to bone health. But vitamin D doesn't act alone—the maintenance of strong, healthy bones is an example of the synergy between vitamin A, vitamin D, and calcium. Vitamin D acts as a hormone within our bodies, and hormones are messengers that tell the body what to do with raw materials. One of vitamin D's critical roles is enabling our bodies to absorb and use calcium properly, and, in concert with vitamin A, this keeps our bones healthy. Fancy, right?

Our girl Gwyneth Paltrow, who has inspired countless others to follow her lead in diet and lifestyle, began supplementing with vitamin D and was told by her doctors to spend time in the sun after she was diagnosed with osteopenia, which was likely a result of vitamin D levels that were "the lowest [her doctors] had ever seen." Osteopenia, a condition of lowered bone density that is considered a harbinger for osteoporosis, occurs in part due to lowered vitamin D status.

That Gwyneth was told to supplement with vitamin D is no surprise, but her doctors' recommendation that she get some good, old-fashioned sunshine may come as a shock. Although we know that vitamin D is synthesized within our bodies through the action of the sun on our skin—that's why hippies like me call it the "sunshine vitamin"—we've also been taught, at least since sunscreen lotions hit the mass market, that the sun is dangerous.

We didn't always think this way. In the late 1800s and early 1900s, before supplements became the preferred way to bolster vitamin D status, a vitamin D deficiency disease called rickets, which affects bone development in children, was treated with a combination of sun exposure and vitamin D–rich foods, like eggs, lard, milk, and cod liver oil (incidentally, these foods are also rich in vitamin A). Rickets occurred frequently during this period, a consequence of industrialization: new, tall buildings and smog blocked the sun and thus vitamin D production in the body. But because it predated both our fear of the cholesterol-rich foods that carry vitamin D and our all-encompassing fear of the sun, the treatment was not so controversial as it might sound to our modern ears.

Rickets was all but eradicated in the United States by the 1930s, but we're seeing a reappearance of vitamin D–related bone disorders in our modern world. Osteopenia, osteoporosis, and a resurgence of rickets are all associated with the same old-is-new-again problem: dysfunction in calcium metabolism and utilization brought on by underlying vitamin D deficiency.

Bones and vitamin D. You get it. But here's the interesting thing: Vitamin D doesn't just affect our bones. We now know that depression, high blood pressure, autism, acne, psoriasis, diabetes, obesity, multiple sclerosis, preeclampsia, heart disease, fibromyalgia, inflammatory bowel disease, other autoimmune diseases, and many forms of cancer are all associated with vitamin D deficiency.

Vitamin D deficiency is a silent epidemic that affects both adults and children in ways we may not even grasp yet.

Here's where things get intense: Vitamin D–deficiency diseases and deficiency-associated health problems may have reemerged today as a consequence of several so-called health movements of the last several decades—first, the heart disease–related fear of cholesterol-containing foods, which also happen to be the foods richest in vitamin D, like eggs, cod liver oil, and lard; and second, the habitual avoidance of the sun's rays, which stimulate vitamin D production inside the body. These changes, in retrospect, were a recipe for widespread vitamin D deficiency.

Many adults today—members of the first sun-fearing generations who have spent most of their lives avoiding natural sources of vitamin D—are clinically deficient in vitamin D and totally unaware of it. The children of this sun-fearing parental generation, who have been slathered in sunscreen since babyhood, are lined up for deficiency from the beginning. And breast-feeding infants, even though they're receiving the most nutritious food possible, are still vulnerable to the consequences of maternal vitamin D deficiency—if Mom doesn't have enough vitamin D, it can have devastating consequences for the infant's bone development and long-term health.

It's actually not surprising that vitamin D deficiency would take its toll on our health in so many ways, because our bodies are designed to work with a robust supply of vitamin D that they just aren't getting. Every cell in our bodies, from top to tail and face to feet, has vitamin D receptors. This means that every single cell uses vitamin D—for example, the brain uses vitamin D for cognitive tasks, the immune system uses vitamin D to stimulate the generation of T cells, and vitamin D can serve as a broad-function antioxidant. When we're deficient, our bodies suffer the consequences.

Our need for vitamin D makes perfect sense in the bright light of evolution. The importance of vitamin D—in particular, vitamin D derived from the sun—is a story that spans both history and biology and, of course, includes a good dose of controversy. Given what we've been told about the danger of the sun's rays, this may be impossible to believe, but here's the truth: Our fear of the sun, not the sun itself, could be what's really hurting us.

Hear me out.

Remember, the whole Paleo concept isn't just about food. It's about learning from our ancestors and adopting modern interpretations of the behaviors that kept them healthy. It's about connecting modern science with hundreds and thousands and millions of years of history. Much of this has to do with chow. But it also has to do with the environment we evolved in.

It makes sense that our cells are wired with vitamin D receptors, and it's no accident that vitamin D plays a profound role in human health. Why? Because we evolved with the sun, in the sun, and because of the sun. Humans evolved near the equator, where sunlight is abundant. Sunlight literally powered our evolution: In the first vertebrates, our most distant ancestors, vitamin D from the sun worked together with calcium to develop the bone matrix. Cool, right?

Today, vitamin D remains important to every cell in our bodies. And it may not just be vitamin D but all the other coproducts the body produces during the creation of sunlight-derived vitamin D that are critical.

That's why we can't let our conditioned fear of sunlight lead us to choose supplements instead of sunshine, or even to rely solely on food for vitamin D. Although we can get it from some foods (and some mighty Paleo ones at that), only the sun gives us health-promoting coproducts alongside vitamin D—including sulfate, which protects the skin from ultraviolet damage, strengthens the immune system, helps prevent cancer and heart disease, and helps the body process toxins; and melanin, an antioxidant that can destroy DNA-damaging free radicals. Ten more beneficial coproducts of vitamin D synthesis are also generated thanks to the sun's action on our skin, none of which we can get from food or supplements. By enjoying the phenomenal, free gift of sunshine, we're actually banking nutrients. For a lazy goof like me, that's a fabulous return on investment.

Yet when we think of the sun, the negative associations are immediate. We love it, but it's dangerous. It enables us to go about our lives, but it's bad for us. Our entire existence is dependent on the sun, but it's going to hurt us—maybe even kill us. We're told that not even a little bit is safe and that we should slather on sunscreen daily. God forbid we walk from our homes to our cars with exposed, unprotected skin.

It's true that sun exposure could be a powerful determinant in our potential for cancer, but not in the way we might think. Vitamin D deficiency has been linked with colon, breast, ovarian, cervical, pancreatic, prostate, and bladder cancers, and more evidence is mounting for its role in the development of other cancers as well.

But what about skin cancer?

It's true that excessive exposure to UV light can damage the skin, causing photoaging and, with long-term overexposure, cancer. Yet it's also true that vitamin D from the sun is absolutely critical to our health, including for the prevention of cancer, and foods and supplements just can't do what the sun can. How do we reconcile these facts?

With information. Our beliefs about the sun, skin cancer, and sunscreen are well intentioned but, in all likelihood, harmful to our health. For the whole sun story, we need to get a bird's-eye view. The controversial part: The vitamin D–deficiency dilemma has an easy solution—responsible sun exposure—but it's one we're both afraid of and biased against. The multibillion-dollar sunscreen industry was built on our fear of the sun.

The truth about sun exposure, vitamin D, and cancer—especially skin cancer—has been in the shadows for far too long. Let's shed a little light on the truth.

The sun's rays, skin cancer, and sunscreen

We blame the sun for skin cancer, but it's not that simple. If it were, our years of slathering sunscreen and avoiding the sun would have resulted in a decrease in skin cancer diagnoses. But since sun protection factor (SPF) sunscreens received FDA approval in the 1970s, the incidence of melanoma in children has risen nearly 3 percent per year—throughout the 1970s and 1980s, the incidence of melanoma in the United States increased faster than that of any other cancer. Since the 1960s, rates of skin cancer in lighter-skinned populations—those at highest risk for skin cancer—have continued to increase by between 5 and 8 percent every single year. First-time melanoma diagnoses overall have tripled over the past thirty-five years, and just between 2000 and 2013 there was a nearly 2 percent increase each year.

But despite all that, rather than questioning what we think we know about the sun and skin cancer, we retreat further into our beliefs. We slather on more sunscreen. We wonder why the dermatologist had to remove that mole when we "did everything right."

It's because we haven't been doing *anything* right.

The recent rise in skin cancer—despite the sunscreen industry's selling enough "protection" to yield billion-dollar profits—is made more puzzling by the typical modern lifestyle: We're hardly ever in the sun. Indoor "screen time" has replaced many outdoor activities. Instead of playing football in the yard, we play virtual football on the PlayStation; instead of going out to the ball game, we watch it on TV. Instead of going for a walk with friends, we text and tweet. We gather our vegetables from fluorescent-lit supermarkets rather than sun-drenched outdoor gardens, for cryin' out loud. We're inside, away from the sun, far more than we were in the past—heck, most of us have jobs that keep us inside when the sun's out.

Oddly enough, working indoors has actually been shown to accompany an *increased* risk of melanoma in several studies. One study of indoor workers observed a steadily increasing rate of malignant melanoma even though the workers were exposed to as much as nine times *less* sunlight than outdoor workers, whose rates of malignant melanoma have not increased. These studies concluded that sun exposure actually helps protect against skin cancer, thanks to the vitamin D generated in the body as a result of sun exposure.

Understanding the sun's ultraviolet (UV) rays will help us understand all this. To this point I've talked a bit about UVB rays, which stimulate vitamin D production in our bodies. It's important to understand UVB, but there's another ray that's equally important to know about: UVA.

UVA rays penetrate the skin more deeply than UVB rays, and only UVB rays stimulate the production of melanin. Melanin, which also causes us to tan, protects our bodies from UV-induced damage by scattering solar radiation and acting as an antioxidant. Once UV exposure has exceeded melanin's ability to protect us, our skin begins to redden and develop inflammation—otherwise known as sunburn. The cascade from tanning to burning is prompted by UVB rays, and this is why they are known as "burning rays." Habitual overexposure to UVB rays resulting in chronic sunburns can, over time, contribute to melanoma risk. However, UVB rays are more generally associated with nonmelanoma skin cancer.

We can think of a sunburn as a blessing in disguise: It's a signal that we need to get out of the sun or risk skin damage, and hopefully it leads us to reduce future sun exposure so that it doesn't happen again. (That's called *living and learning*.) Perhaps UVB rays should be called "signal rays" instead of "burning rays." UVB signal rays help warn us when we're in danger of overexposure and the skin damage that comes with it, usually starting with that hint of pink on fairer skin. UVA rays offer no such warning.

UVA rays penetrate into the deeper layers of the skin and can cause more damage to skin cells than UVB rays. UVA rays cause oxidative damage, which can lead to photoaging, including wrinkles and collagen loss. Worse yet, UVA rays can damage our DNA. UVA does not cause us to tan or burn as UVB does; in fact, it actually causes damage to our melanin-producing cells—which is why it is associated with malignant melanoma, the deadliest form of skin cancer. Since UVA rays don't give us that sunburn signal, they can wreak havoc and leave no immediate trace.

Here's the most important distinction between UVB and UVA rays: Sunscreen easily blocks UVB rays and their effects, including sunburn, cancer-fighting vitamin D, and the antioxidant melanin. UVB rays are also blocked by windows. UVA rays are not blocked by either windows or sunscreen.

This means that we're exposed to damaging UVA rays without the benefit of sunburn to tell us when we've had enough. Whether we're sitting indoors near a window, in a car with the sun streaming through the windshield, or on a beach slathered in SPF 35, we're soaking up excessive amounts of UVA.

So is sunscreen protecting us at all? Not really, although there's a time and a place for certain other types of sun protection, as we'll discuss.

Sunscreen is rated according to its SPF, which stands for "sun protection factor." The concept was first approved by the FDA in the 1970s for use in the marketing of sunscreen. SPF rates only the sunscreen's ability to block UVB, not UVA, rays; the measure was developed as a means of avoiding UVB-induced sunburn—before we knew just how damaging UVA rays could be. Thanks to sunscreen, we thought we were free to spend hours upon hours in the sun, and we believed that because we weren't burning, we were A-OK.

What sunscreen has done is not so much protect us as lull us into a false sense of security while opening the door to damage that would never occur if we were able to heed our bodies' natural warning signals.

When we block UVB rays while keeping the door open to UVA rays, thinking we're protected because we aren't getting burned, we allow the most damaging rays to penetrate our skin and do their insidious work, even as we block our burn signal and stop the production of melanin and cancer-preventing, immune-boosting vitamin D. This may leave us more vulnerable to cancer than ever before.

So-called broad-spectrum sunscreens, which claim to protect against both UVB and UVA rays, attempt to combine SPF-based UVB protection with chemicals meant to absorb or disperse UVA rays. However, the Environmental Working Group cautions that broad-spectrum sunscreens sold in the United States are produced according to FDA criteria that are "the weakest in the modern world." In Europe, broad-spectrum sunscreens must provide UVA protection at least one-third as potent as its UVB protection. In the United States, not a single broad-spectrum sunscreen meets even this minimally effective criterion. Most of us think that when we choose a broad-spectrum sunscreen, our UVA protection matches the SPF. This is absolutely not the case. To add insult to injury, many of these sunscreens contain retinyl palmitate, a chemical found by the FDA to increase the growth rate of skin tumors.

Sunscreen lotions were a good idea in theory, but, to put it nicely, they just never panned out. Because we were concerned about the dangers of the sun's rays yet ill-informed about which rays helped and which ones harmed, we created sunscreen technology that actually interferes with our own biology instead of helping us protect ourselves. We've gone so far down the rabbit hole of SPFs and broad-spectrum protection and FDA approval that we've forgotten that, just fifty years ago, we had lower rates of skin cancer and exceedingly simple ways of protecting ourselves.

Dermatologist and vitamin D researcher Michael Holick writes, "There is evidence to link sun exposure and vitamin D to every facet of medicine and health." Vitamin D and all the incredible coproducts that our bodies generate from sunshine are critical. They keep our bones healthy and combat chronic disease. They boost our immune system and our mood. They even stimulate the economy—who takes a vacation to get *out* of the sun?

Skin cancer can develop as a result of excessive sun exposure, and it can happen with or without sunscreen; but the type of sun exposure that makes us vulnerable to cancer is vastly different from the type of sun exposure that boosts our vitamin D levels and helps prevent cancer and other maladies.

Most of us are getting too little sunlight, not too much. What we need is *responsible* sun exposure.

Responsible sun exposure: Is there such a thing?

It's a far different thing to look like a cast member of *Jersey Shore* or a piece of tanned leather than it is to have healthy levels of sun-stimulated vitamin D. The good news is, the alternative to sunscreen is not frying, fist-pumping on the boardwalk, or getting cancer. It's simply informed, conscientious, responsible sun exposure.

Like *Desperate Housewives* reunion specials and music by the Eagles, when it comes to the sun, a little can go a long way.

How does this work? Let's start with the basics: Get sun, but don't burn. You've got that UVB burn signal for a reason, but the best burn signal is the one that never gets used.

Vitamin D–generating UVB rays aren't available year-round in all places. The "vitamin D winter" hits varying parts of the world at different times of the year, usually coinciding with *actual* winter, when we don't want to be outside much anyway. This means that we don't have to worry about getting a daily dose of vitamin D every day of the year. Summertime is usually the best time to boost vitamin D levels, and it can be done in just a few minutes each day. And it can be accomplished simply by *being outside* and getting some sun on your extremities. Go fly a kite!

Each of us can tolerate a different amount of sun before burning. Different skin types and tones tolerate sun exposure differently: People with fair skin can often tolerate very little sun before burning, while those with darker skin tones have a greater degree of built-in sun tolerance because they have more melanin.

Here's the cool part: Those who burn easily require very little sun to generate adequate vitamin D. Minutes of sun exposure at a time will often suffice. Those who do not burn easily will need a bit more sun exposure to generate their vitamin D. These are actually pretty incredible adaptations. Think about it: Over millions of years, as some humans migrated from the equator to northerly regions with far less sun and longer periods of vitamin D winter, their bodies had to adapt to ensure that they could generate enough vitamin D to stay healthy, even when vitamin D from the sun was slim pickin's. These northerners adapted to have less melanin and thus skin that was more sensitive to the sun and produced vitamin D more quickly. Further, as the miracle of nature would have it, abundant cold-water fish, rich in vitamin D, became a dietary staple of northern cultures, which helps compensate for that vitamin D winter. Those incredibly fair-skinned individuals who simply aren't adapted to tolerate a lot of sun are likely adapted to get more vitamin D from food like oily fish, cod liver oil, eggs, and lard.

Another lesson of history and biology: Nature provides everything we need to be healthy, whoever we are and wherever we come from. That said, many of us live in parts of the world where sun exposure doesn't accord with our skin tone. Darker-skinned people living in northerly climates are more prone to vitamin D deficiency, and those with very fair skin living closer to the equator have the highest rates of skin cancer. That's a bit of a bummer, especially for people of northern descent living in, say, Miami; but that's nature for ya. She's always providing, but she doesn't care that you want to spend your summer in a thong in South Beach.

And here's where the "responsible" part of "responsible sun exposure" *really* comes in: When it's time to get out of the sun, *get out of the sun.* The way to protect ourselves from overexposure isn't much different than the way our ancestors did thousands of years in the past: Cover up or find some shade.

There is a middle ground between burning and clothes-wearing or shade-seeking, and that's physical sunblock, the alter-ego of conventional sunscreens. It's that adorable, thick, white cream called zinc oxide that physically blocks rays rather than attempting to absorb or scatter them, much as an article of clothing would. The downside: It's like white body paint. The upside: Once you put it on, you have absolute power to embarrass your friends, mortify your children, and give everyone a really good laugh.

To further protect your skin from damage, dietary strategies are key. An anti-inflammatory diet can heal skin damage and reverse photoaging. Dietary antioxidants both protect the skin from and can reverse damage from overexposure to UV rays. This is where all the nutrient-dense foods I advocate come in: Cholesterol is a powerful antioxidant, as are the fat-soluble vitamins A, D, and K_2. I've talked about cholesterol in depth, along with two of these vitamins, and there's one more left—another critical vitamin that works with vitamins A and D to keep us healthy and happy. That's vitamin K_2.

Nutrients we need:
K$_2$ is for *kick-ass*

....

There's less to say about K$_2$ than there is to say about vitamin A or D, but it's no less important. It's just less well known, so there's less dogma to dismantle.

Have you heard of vitamin K$_2$? Until a few years ago, I sure hadn't. I'd never seen it on a nutrition label; I'd never heard a celebrity talk about it; and it definitely wasn't in any of the "fat-burning" supplements I was taking (ugh, don't get me started). Despite the fact that I was convinced I knew it all, I knew nothing about K$_2$. But that doesn't mean I didn't need it.

If any nutrient can prove to us that we know far less about the many amazing compounds in real foods than we think, it's vitamin K$_2$.

The nutrients we need aren't always the ones on our radar. Sure, as kids we knew that calcium builds strong bones and vitamin C is the reason fruit is good for us; and as adults we're bombarded with news of the latest berry, tea, or extract that promises life-altering effects (although we don't *need* those; on the contrary, we *need* to keep our money and steer clear of the trends). But what about the nutrients that kept humans healthy for centuries before our era of health dogma and nutrition-in-a-capsule? What nutrients did our ancestors eat that we might be missing today?

We've covered the much-maligned vitamins A and D, two nutrients rich in the foods highly valued by our ancestors that, unlike K$_2$, we've known about since the early 1900s. Vitamin A was officially identified in 1906, followed by vitamin D in 1922, so at least those nutrients have had some recognition—even if, at times, it's been unfairly negative press. As any Hollywood starlet would say, it doesn't matter what they're saying as long as they're talking about you.

Nobody was talking about vitamin K_2, though, until around 1940; and even then scientists weren't sure exactly what it was or what to call it. They just knew that it had the power to do amazing things, like prevent tooth decay and heart disease, enable the development of a wide palate and excellent dentition, and contribute to reproductive health. Vitamin K_1 had been identified around 1930, but it didn't have any of the effects of what we now know to be K_2. This is because K_1, which is found in plants, is actually converted into K_2 by the animals that eat those plants, and this conversion gives K_2 its unique, astonishing properties. This wasn't known for many decades after the discovery of K_1, however, so the nutrient remained a mystery. Weston Price called it "Activator X," and though many tried to identify it, it wasn't until 1997 that scientists realized that vitamin K_2 was a unique compound, related to but distinct from vitamin K_1. Nearly ten years after that, in 2006, the USDA finally officially quantified the vitamin K_2 content in foods.

Vitamin K_2 exists in two forms: form K_2 MK-4 and form K_2 MK-7. These are real science terms, not titles of Tom Cruise movies, and they are different variations of the same nutrient—similar enough to bear the same first name, but different enough that they don't have identical effects. Form K_2 MK-7 is derived from bacteria in a traditional Japanese dish called *natto,* a fermented soybean food that is known for its slimy texture and offensive smell. Fortunately for you, this isn't the form I want to talk about.

The form I'm talking about, form K_2 MK-4—hereafter I'll just call it K_2—is found in the tissues and fats of ruminant animals, particularly in their milk fat, and in egg yolks and fish eggs—all foods that fell out of favor, along with nutrients like vitamins A and D, when our modern nutrition dogma took root.

And wouldn't you know it? Vitamin K_2 never acts alone. According to Masterjohn, its effects are dependent on vitamins A and D doing their jobs, signaling cells to produce molecules that vitamin K_2 then activates for a whole down-stream cascade of health-promoting reactions. Synergy strikes again.

Vitamin K_2 deficiency is associated with osteoporosis, heart disease, cancer, diabetes, wrinkles, cavities, and poor dentition and jaw formation. One of K_2's primary responsibilities is to make sure that calcium is deposited in the right places within the body, which is a big deal: Calcification of the arteries is part of the pathology of heart disease, so keeping calcium out of the arteries is critical.

This is all particularly meaningful given our discussion of heart disease in the chapter on fat. In all the decades we've been blaming cholesterol and saturated fat for the growing epidemic of cardiovascular disease, including arterial calcification and blockage, while searching for a magic bullet to prevent it, vitamin K_2—already present in real, traditional food—may have been part of the answer.

Vitamin K_2 is so powerful, says Masterjohn, that "Research is in fact rapidly redefining heart disease largely as a deficiency of this vitamin."

Vitamin K_2's role in calcium distribution also affects the formation of our bones and teeth, which are built with calcium. The development of a wide palate and jaw with plenty of room for all our teeth is largely dependent on vitamin K_2, as well as vitamins A and D. Deficiency in vitamin K_2 can manifest in problems with dental crowding—a common complaint and the backbone of modern orthodontics. Seriously, what kid hasn't had a mouthful of braces? That's all due to K_2. In the same way that maternal vitamin D deficiency can affect the development of a child even before birth, so can K_2 help determine the health of both mother and baby.

This vitamin is so incredible, it leaves me wondering what other amazing, undiscovered nutrients are hidden in real food that we haven't even discovered yet. (As Navin Johnson said, "If this is out there, think how much *more* is out there!")

The creation of vitamin K_2 in animal tissues is yet another example of animals' ability to convert nutrients from plants into more potent nutrients that humans can use. The conversion of vitamin K_1 to vitamin K_2 occurs when ruminant animals eat K_1-rich plants, convert K_1 to K_2 inside their bodies, and concentrate this nutrient in their tissues, fat, and milk. But that conversion can only happen under certain circumstances. Ruminant animals must be grazing on growing green plants—as in, those plants must be attached to the ground just as Mother Nature intended, and the healthier the soil in which those plants grow, the better. Being a meat-eater means demanding the soil is cared for and the plant kingdom is respected, even if the plants aren't going directly into our mouths. Unsurprisingly, you won't find appreciable vitamin K_2 in conventional meats or milk. It's the conscientious farmer raising animals on well-tended pasture, not the CAFO, who holds the key to vitamin K_2–rich food.

Vitamin K_2 is concentrated in high amounts in milk fat, in part because it's so critical for the healthy growth and development of newborn mammals (including humans). One of the many reasons I absolutely love butter and ghee from grass-fed cows—aside from the fact that they're delicious—is that they're rich in the critical fat-soluble vitamins, and they're two of our best sources of vitamin K_2.

If you're just not into dairy, you can still find vitamin K_2 in organ meats, like liver; egg yolks from properly raised hens; and fish eggs. However you get it, I highly suggest you seek it out, and from food, not supplements. All the foods rich in vitamin K_2 are also rich in many other nutrients, and these nutrients work together in a way that a lab-created supplement just can't match.

Nutrients we need: Omega-3 (or, fish oil—what's the catch?)

By this point you may have noticed two recurring themes: Creatures concentrate and convert the nutrition found in plants into forms humans can best use; and supplements can't replicate the synergy of nutrients found together in real food. Nowhere is this more relevant than with omega-3, including the omega-3 found in fish oil.

First, an important distinction: Fish oil supplements, a highly processed source of omega-3 with just a few decades of history behind it, are completely different from the cod liver oil I've referred to previously. Cod liver oil has been a staple health food in several cultures, including our own, for centuries, and it provides a concentrated source of vitamins A and D with trace amounts of naturally occurring omega-3. (Unfortunately, companies that produce cod liver oil in keeping with traditional methods that preserve nutrient content are scarce, but they're out there.)

Swimming—er, moving *right* along.

When you read the words *fish oil,* did you think about the oil in whole fish or the oil in supplement capsules?

If you thought of the oil in supplement capsules, you're in good company. The precious omega-3 fatty acids found in oily cold-water fish—eicosapentaenoic acid (EPA) and docosahexaenoic acid (DHA)—are the liquid gold that drives the fish oil supplement industry. And because our culture is saturated with supplements and the obsessive search for that more-is-better magic bullet, we're more inclined to go crazy for a capsule than we are to, ya know, just eat more omega-3-rich fish. I had fish oil capsules shipped to my house every ninety days for a good year before I ever considered cracking open a tin of sardines. I sure wasn't alone: Americans spent more than $1 billion on fish oil supplements in 2010.

We go bubbles for EPA and DHA, and for good reason: They are profoundly anti-inflammatory. The body uses them to generate signaling molecules called *eicosanoids* that keep the immune system calm. They are critical for eye health, brain health, infant brain development, and reproductive health, and they are associated with a reduced risk of cardiovascular disease—the holy grail of health benefits.

Because of these remarkable—and highly marketable—effects, the term *omega-3* has become an incredibly lucrative one. The global market for foods fortified with omega-3 has reached $25 billion. Companies are starting to put omega-3 in all kinds of stuff: It's a staple in multivitamins, and it's even added to granola bars and margarine. The taglines "rich in omega-3!" and "a good source of omega-3!" are incredibly profitable.

This commercial marketability—and the omega-3 marketers' propensity for phraseology—should make us slightly suspicious. What's the catch?

The catch is this: When we see the term *omega-3*, it doesn't necessarily refer to the critically important EPA and DHA, though we've been led to believe that all omega-3s are the same (they're not). There are actually different types of omega-3, and to reap the health benefits we hear about, we need the right kind, from the right sources, and in the right amounts. It shouldn't come from plants, and it shouldn't come from fortified foods or supplements.

Actually, that's more than one catch. Thoroughly confused? Are things starting to smell . . . fishy?

When it comes to nutrients, omega-3 is among the most misunderstood. Let's fix that, starting with a little chat about what omega-3 is in the first place.

Most people think that omega-3 and EPA and DHA are one and the same, and that any omega-3 is good omega-3. This belief has been profitable for many omega-3 purveyors, but there's more to the story.

Omega-3 refers to a class of polyunsaturated fatty acid, of which there are several types. Two of those types, and the types with the most profound health benefits, are EPA and DHA. These are abundant in oily cold-water fish. (DHA is also found in algae and is sent up the food chain through the fish that eat it.) When we talk about fish oil supplements, we're actually talking about encapsulated EPA and DHA, refined from whole fish. Yes, *refined* is still a dirty word—even when it comes to fish oil. We'll get to that.

Another type of omega-3, alpha-linolenic acid (ALA), is a short-chain omega-3 found in plants and plant oils that we humans sometimes eat, like flax, flax oil, nuts, nut oils, and canola (blech); and plants that animals eat, like leaves and grass. ALA is the omega-3 often used to fortify foods, usually in the form of a refined ALA-rich oil. If you're told that a plant or plant oil is "rich in omega-3"—a common justification for the much-advertised "health benefits" of trendy foods like flax or junky industrial products like canola oil—it's not the type of omega-3 we actually want. It's not EPA or DHA.

This doesn't mean that all foods containing ALA are unhealthy—nuts and seeds are whole, perfectly nutritious foods, and many of the pricier, cold-pressed nut oils are fine and dandy on occasion—but they're not sources of EPA or DHA. In the case of refined crop oils rich in ALA, however, there's that pesky problem of being, ya know, highly processed devil spawn.

Despite the fact that EPA and DHA are the omega-3s we need most, ALA remains a source of nutritional confusion, in part because it is the only omega-3 that is biologically "essential." When we hear the word *essential*, we think, "I must absolutely need that, like I need a black blazer or a DVD box set of Season 1 of *The O.C.* (you know, for posterity)." However, in nutrition, *essential* doesn't mean "absolutely necessary"; it simply means "the body can't manufacture this itself, so if we want it, we must get it from food." The fact that it's "essential" has nothing to do with how important ALA is to our bodies; in fact, ALA's most redeeming quality is that it can be converted (albeit not very well) to the omega-3s we absolutely do need: EPA and DHA.

Indeed, our bodies can convert ALA to EPA, and from there, EPA can be converted into DHA, which is the final, end-usable form of omega-3. These omega-3s exist on a sort of continuum, beginning with ALA and ending with DHA. Until it is converted, the health benefits of ALA cannot match the health benefits of EPA and DHA. Unfortunately, like the body's ability to convert beta-carotene to vitamin A, the body's ability to convert ALA to EPA and then to DHA is extremely poor—by some accounts, less than 1 percent of ALA ends up as DHA, and even the most generous estimates top out at around 10 percent. This is a terrible, horrible, no good, very bad rate of return. It would require extreme, excessive intake of ALA to meet the body's basic requirements for DHA.

Yet we need EPA and DHA, so we've got to get it somehow. Many vegans and vegetarians are told that, because of the body's ability to convert ALA into EPA and DHA, it's not necessary to obtain EPA or DHA from fish. This represents much of the confusion around our understanding of omega-3s—and it could present a danger to those counting on the pitiful ALA conversion rate. To further compound the vegan dilemma, the conversion of ALA to EPA and DHA requires enzymes that depend on animal-derived nutrients such as saturated fat, biotin, and vitamin B_6.

So: The EPA and DHA found in oily cold-water fish, and all so-called fish oils, are omega-3s, but not all omega-3s are EPA and DHA, and they certainly don't all carry the same benefits. Got it?

To make things even more confusing, EPA and DHA are not found exclusively in fish. While oily fish are the richest whole-creature sources of EPA and DHA, ruminant animals can convert ALA from grass and leaves into EPA and DHA, much as they convert beta-carotene to true vitamin A, although the amount of EPA and DHA in ruminant animal tissues is low compared to the amount of EPA and DHA in oily fish. While the smidge of EPA and DHA is a bonus on top of all the other great things about properly raised meats, it's not the main benefit.

Which is why oily fish are the ideal source of EPA and DHA. They're simply the best, better than all the rest. They take your heart and make it stronger, baby—on top of all their other health benefits, of course.

But oily fish aren't the best only because of their omega-3 content. It's also because of the fish itself. I wasn't surprised to learn that the study that sparked the omega-3 frenzy looked at people who ate not lots of fish oil supplements but lots of *fish*. Researchers concluded that the benefits these people seemed to reap from eating oily fish were a result of EPA and DHA, but oily fish is also rich in other extraordinary nutrients that could've played a part, such as whole protein, vitamin D, selenium, iodine, and taurine. These nutrients benefit the heart, the body's detoxification systems, hormonal balance, and even skin and hair. It's possible, then, that all these nutrients were the true cause of the benefits that were originally attributed to EPA and DHA alone.

The lead researcher of a recent study questioning the benefits of fish oil supplements suggested that perhaps we should just eat more whole fish. This study found that fish oil supplementation does not reduce deaths from any cause, including cardiovascular disease. This doesn't mean that fish oil won't benefit anyone ever, but it certainly doesn't seem to be as beneficial as we've been led to believe. Real food wins again.

So fish oil supplements, which are composed solely of isolated EPA and DHA that have been processed out of whole fish, carry none of the other amazing nutrients found in whole fish. That's a bummer. A bigger bummer: As discussed in the chapter on fat, polyunsaturated fats, including omega-3s, are quite fragile. Not only does extracting them from their natural protective packaging—the fish itself—make them vulnerable to damage, but the very process of extraction is no better than the harsh process of refining industrial crop oils.

The oil in fish oil supplements isn't squeezed out of the fish and right into your supplement bottle. The fish mass must be heated so that the proteins coagulate, rupturing fat stores and allowing the oil to be separated and pressed out. Then, after the oil is pressed out of the fish, it must be chemically refined, neutralized with acid, separated and washed multiple times, and finally encapsulated and shipped off to your friendly local supplement store. Oh, and just as in the crop oil industry, the by-product fish protein is often sold off as animal feed.

That's not the only argument against fish oil supplements. Thanks to our modern, more-is-better mind-set, we tend to think that we need a clinical crap-ton of fish oil to be healthy; therefore, the habitual pill-swallowing and guzzling of liquid fish oil supplements is commonplace. This actually does more harm than good. (Stop it. Stop it right now.)

The problems with fish oil supplements are the problems with most supplements. First, isolating and sucking down supplemental nutrients makes it far too easy to go overboard on those nutrients and surpass our bodies' actual need for them, which is better served by whole foods. Second, isolating and sucking down nutrients without thought for the *other* nutrients that, in nature, occur alongside them means throwing off the natural nutrient balance that real, whole, nutrient-rich food imparts to our bodies. Nutrient synergy, remember?

Our bodies' requirement for omega-3 is actually relatively low. We need no more than we can get from whole, nutrient-rich foods, including whole seafood and properly raised animal foods.

Here's where it gets more interesting. Not only is our requirement for omega-3 relatively low, as only a small, predetermined amount can be incorporated into a healthy cell membrane, but it's also important to keep omega-3 DHA in proper balance with its complementary nutrient, omega-6 arachidonic acid (AA).

Much like omega-3, omega-6 exists on a continuum, which begins with so-called essential linoleic acid (LA)—which is abundant in plants, especially crop oils like corn and canola (again, blech)—and progresses to arachidonic acid and beyond. Arachidonic acid is the omega-6 fat we most need (I'll get to that). Like the conversion of ALA to DHA, the conversion of LA to AA is unreliable, and it depends on nutrients (biotin and vitamin B_6) that are abundant in animal products—which poses a problem for plants-only eaters. Fortunately, however, as with omega-3 DHA, we don't have to rely on that conversion process to get our AA. We can get it from animal foods like organ meats and egg yolks, no conversion necessary. (I'll take any opportunity to bring the conversation back to egg yolks.)

Yes, we *need* omega-6 AA. Popular diet books and buzz have propagated the notion that omega-6 AA is "bad" and inflammatory, and that less is best. However, the truth is that omega-6 AA is as important as omega-3 DHA. Like omega-3s, omega-6 fats are used to form eicosanoids that drive the proper function of the immune system. Where omega-3 DHA has anti-inflammatory effects, AA initiates the inflammation process that enables our bodies to heal themselves and repair damage as necessary. DHA and AA have complementary jobs, and their relationship is synchronistic, not antagonistic.

At least, it should be. Guess how we can mess up that natural balance? By eating crappy foods instead of whole, nourishing foods, and by overdoing the supplements. In other words: by trying to be smarter than real food.

For example, when we eat too many highly processed, LA-rich crop oils—as modern nutritional guidelines encourage us to do—omega-6 can begin competing with omega-3, and they stop working together and start working against one another. Factory-farmed animals that eat the same crop-based crud also end up with too much omega-6 in their tissues, a problem that's passed along to us if we eat them (in contrast to properly raised creatures eating their natural diets, which concentrate omega-3 and omega-6 in the appropriate levels and ratios). A chronic excess of omega-6 sets the stage for out-of-control inflammation, which further inhibits the conversion of "essential" omega-3 and omega-6 to the forms we actually need, and it keeps any DHA and AA within our bodies from being utilized properly.

On the flip side, any omega-3 supplement, including plant oils, fish oils, or algae-based DHA—a vegan-friendly DHA source—can end up outcompeting the synthesis of arachidonic acid as well. Sigh. Can we win at this game? (Yes, Virginia.)

The end-goal of much of the supplementation and exhausting omega-3 and omega-6 bean-counting is generally to balance the ratios of omega-3 to omega-6 in our diet. It's a noble idea, and not without precedent: Ancestral hunter-gatherer diets are estimated to have contained one unit of omega-3 for every one to four units of omega-6, in contrast to the one-to-twenty (and higher), massively pro-inflammatory ratios of today. What we often forget, however, is that the ideal, balanced hunter-gatherer ratios were achieved through the free eating of real, whole foods.

Isn't that always what it comes back to? Eat real food, and let the chips fall . . . into perfect alignment?

Unfortunately, the simplest roads to getting healthier have been totally overshadowed by profit-driven industries, supplement crazes, and deeply ingrained myths that make the simple truth sound just—what—too darn easy? Though I could talk about this stuff all day, from myths to glorious truths, in the end all ya need to do is eat some friggin' sardines and some frackin' egg yolks, and you're good to go.

Forget the ratios and the bean-counting and the nitpicking and focus on real food for your omega goodness. Don't guzzle fish oil like it's going out of style. We don't need fish oil supplements—we need fish and the omega-3 abundance of the sea, along with the nourishment of omega-6-rich egg yolks and properly raised animal foods, and less of the junk that interferes with our efforts to get healthy. Don't like fish? I'm sorry, that distaste won't magically make fish oil less processed or more safe. It won't insert selenium, iodine, and taurine into junky plant oils. I resolved to love sardines, and at some point, I realized I actually *did* love them. Even more so, I loved the health benefits I could see and feel that I never got from fish oil. You can do it.

Nutrients we need: Minerals matter, and they're better together

Dietary minerals are chemical elements our bodies require to function at the most basic level, and we need many different types of minerals to be fully healthy. Dietary minerals can be subdivided into two groups: macrominerals and trace minerals.

Both macrominerals and trace minerals are vital to our bodies' abilities to work properly. Our metabolisms require minerals. Our hearts beat and our muscles move and our mouths flap because of them. Our reproductive functions depend on them. Despite all this, we're barely educated about them—except, of course, for a few nuggets of conventional wisdom that have come to comprise the entirety of our modern-day understanding of these critical chemicals.

These morsels of mineral miseducation are all warped in their own special ways. First, we're taught that calcium is the "milk mineral" and that it's critical for us to get lots of it from dairy products. Second, we're taught that salt—a dietary mineral created through the ionic bond of sodium and chlorine, often simply referred to as "sodium" in the nutrition world—should be avoided whenever possible. And third, we're taught (or rather, led to assume) that when it comes to all the other minerals we need . . . well, pay no attention to the man behind that curtain.

Conventional wisdom, as usual, has led us astray.

Calcium controversy?

Remember all the cool celebrities with milk mustaches who have, over the last two decades, encouraged us to drink milk as if our calcium—er, *cool factor* depended on it? The Got Milk campaign, which has featured well-known actors, athletes, and even cartoon characters gettin' their milk mustache on, is a long-running project of the California Milk Processor Board (CMPB), which was established by California's Department of Agriculture. Both the campaign and the CMPB were formed in 1993 to address lagging dairy sales in the 1980s. The campaign worked, so much so that it has continued to run for twenty years.

And by "the campaign worked," I mean that it gave the conventional dairy industry the boost it needed, as evidenced not only by the campaign's longevity but also by the spike in large-scale dairy production operations since the early 1990s. Between 1997 and 2007, the number of small dairy farms in America—the "little guys"—dwindled while the number of dairy cows on large-scale factory farms nearly doubled. This was good for Big Dairy's bottom line, but the benefits end there: Factory farming is not a natural, compassionate, biologically or environmentally appropriate, or necessary way to produce food, let alone healthy food.

Unfortunately, most conventional dairy—that is, the dairy we see on supermarket shelves—comes from those factory farms. The cows are treated poorly, fed unnatural food, and often inundated with growth hormones and nontherapeutic antibiotics. They develop mastitis, among other illnesses, and because of this they often get sick and die quickly. Their milk is homogenized, pasteurized, reconstituted, and fortified, and the products made from this milk are loaded with additives and stabilizers. Calling this kind of dairy a real, whole food is like calling a Twinkie a balanced meal. It's not. It's a processed product.

This is in stark contrast to real milk, which was briefly discussed in the chapter on carbs. Dairy from properly raised animals has a long history in the human diet, and it's actually a very savvy means of getting reliable nutrition. At their best, real, raw dairy products are a natural, nutrient-rich source of crucial vitamins like A, D, and K_2. In its raw, natural state, milk is unpasteurized, unhomogenized, and perfectly safe to drink. Those who can't tolerate raw cow's milk may tolerate raw goat's or sheep's milk, which have also been part of the human diet for thousands of years.

This is a point where I differ from many proponents of a Paleo lifestyle. Many "by-the-bookers" argue that all dairy, regardless of source or quality, is "not Paleo" and thus, by extension, is "bad." If that were sound logic, then anything that wasn't available to a caveman or -woman would be bad: Modern grass-fed beef would be bad, since the oldest known cattle breeds surviving into modern time are only a few thousand years old; modern means of communication would be bad, since Paleolithic folks didn't have cell phones; and modern supermarkets and even farmer's markets would be bad, since Paleo people had to hunt and gather everything they got.

All I'm saying is, don't be so literal that you miss the forest for the trees (or the butter for the list of diet rules). Just get to know your food, how you tolerate it, and the myths behind it, and go for the foods that have a long history and lots of nutrients. This Paleo thing is about outsmarting the hype, not creating new hype.

It's often argued that the scientific evidence against dairy is insurmountable and that, even if it weren't, it makes no sense to consume dairy because no other earthly creature drinks the milk of another species. These contentions are false. While conventional dairy has, in fact, been observed to be intensely problematic in some studies, this is to be expected: Dairy from sick, poorly fed cows in the industrial feedlot system that is processed, defatted, skimmed, and pasteurized is bound to cause problems—it's a processed food. Raw dairy, however, is the polar opposite of this conventional crud, and its proponents swear by its health value. There is very little evidence against real, raw, properly produced milk. Further, when given access to the milk of other species, animals of all species actually *do* take advantage of that nutrition. Predators don't balk at the mammary glands of their prey. The hurdle for most animals is opportunity, and humans, at the top of the food chain, have created the opportunity to enjoy nutrient-dense dairy by developing symbiotic relationships with other animals. A Jersey cow, given shelter and a safe place to pasture, in return gives the farmer nutritious raw milk.

But here's another truth: Just because raw milk is healthful and nutrient-rich doesn't mean that we humans need it. In addition to burying the very important difference between conventional milk and raw milk, another unfortunate consequence of the aggressive, successful marketing of conventional milk is that we continue to believe that milk is a vital, irreplaceable source of calcium. Of course, it makes sense that we're inclined to fret so much about how much calcium we get. Calcium is the most abundant mineral in the body. It makes up our teeth and our skeletons. But there's far more involved in getting the calcium our bodies need than just the amount of calcium we ingest.

In reality, we don't need milk for calcium at all. A cup of conventional whole milk contains 276 mg of calcium. A cup of cooked collard greens has 266 mg. A cup of cooked spinach has 245 mg. Two and a half ounces of sardines—roughly one-half cup—has 284 mg. Bone broth and stock, traditional foods that serve as the base of many culinary creations, from the most complex dish to the most basic soup, are made by simmering animal bones and aromatic vegetables in water and are excellent sources of highly bioavailable calcium— the longer the bones are cooked, the more calcium becomes available.

The U.S. government sets a recommended daily intake (RDI) of over 1,000 mg of calcium daily for the average adult. This number, however, and the government's recommended intake standards in general have been the subject of controversy since the 1980s. Because the nutrient intake recommendations are modeled on the government's dietary recommendations (formerly the Food Pyramid, now MyPlate) and vice versa, they must reflect one another. One hand washes the other, in other words, and these hands are awfully dirty. A 1988 article by a University of Massachusetts nutrition professor titled "Ecology of Food and Nutrition" criticized the development of the intake recommendations, stating that they did not take into account "factors that influence the efficacy of nutrient utilization" (in other words, nutrient synergy). The article warned that the recommendations would undoubtedly decrease as knowledge of this concept evolved. Unfortunately, by 2000, knowledge of nutrient synergy had not evolved at all, and the recommended intake for calcium was specifically called into question in an article published in the *American Journal of Clinical Nutrition* in 2000. This article reiterated that the existing recommended intake guidelines were based on uncertainty and ignorance of the complex role of calcium and other cofactors in maintaining bone density. Calcium is important, but we likely need less calcium and more cofactors.

In summary, hammering the body with calcium does not mean that the body will use it properly. All the milk, milkshakes, and malted milk balls (kidding) on the planet won't guarantee that we have the cofactors needed to allow the body to use the calcium it's given. Natural (not synthetic) vitamins D and K_2—which are both missing in conventional milk—allow the body to absorb and use calcium to maintain healthy bones, and exercise strengthens the bones as well. Calcium's movement across cell membranes, which affects muscle activation, is regulated by magnesium, another cofactor for calcium. Magnesium also activates vitamin D so that it can modulate the absorption of calcium. And a proper balance of fatty acids in the cell membrane is needed for the transmission of minerals across the membranes.

Where are all these cofactors found? In real foods—the same real foods that also contain calcium. In raw milk, meat, seafood, properly made bone broth, and vegetables. Are we sensing a pattern?

It's not just the truth about calcium that has been whitewashed. The truth about salt is also rocky terrain.

Salty situations (or, take what you've been told about salt with a grain of salt)

Chemically, salt is NaCl, or sodium chloride. When dissolved in water, it becomes an important electrolyte that conducts the body's electrical impulses. It's needed for every cell in the human body, from muscle to brain, to function properly. We literally cannot live without salt.

Historically, salt once represented not just health but also wealth and security: The origins of the word *salary* are rooted in the Latin word for salt, which alludes to a time thousands of years in the past when local economies, large and small, were based around the salt trade. Salt was vital for keeping domesticated livestock healthy and preserving foods, and it even served as medicine in early cultures. It was so highly valued that whole civilizations were said to go to war because of it.

Currently, salt is a savory granule of ongoing dietary controversy. It has the honor of being falsely demonized, right alongside saturated fat and cholesterol, in the blame game for heart disease. Specifically, salt is blamed for chronic hypertension thanks, in large part, to less-than-trustworthy dietary recall studies, and chronic hypertension—chronically elevated blood pressure—is a risk factor for heart disease. Many individuals diagnosed with heart disease also happen to suffer from high blood pressure. In the conventional medical and nutrition worlds, this winding road of associations is consolidated into one false belief: that salt intake can cause heart disease, and therefore, we must eat less of it.

Sigh.

The modern campaign against salt, based on this specious science, began in the 1970s and gained momentum through the 1980s. The vitriol now associated with this formerly respectable staple has been enough to all but wipe out thousands of years of historical and biological value.

If salt was so highly valued over thousands of years, and if it's so critical to our bodies, why did it suddenly, just forty years ago, become so reviled? Like most of the modern myths surrounding what we eat and why, this is a story of processing, politics, and misplaced blame.

Today, we often think of salt as "bad," whether we're simply using a pinch for flavor or listing one of many additives found in processed food. Salt is our oldest natural preservative, and it is indeed still used to maintain the shelf life and modulate the flavor of modern processed foods; but in that case, salt is simply a victim of its own usefulness. Hijacked

by the processed-food industry, salt has endured many ma-
nipulations to become as useful as possible in refined junk.
Salt as nature intended, however, is as natural as sunshine.

The salt we eat, no matter where it is found or how it is
collected, originated in the salty sea. Mined from ancient underground deposits or evaporated from seawater, unrefined
salt comes in all shapes, colors, and sizes, thanks to the suite
of other minerals that occur naturally in saltwater and the
regions in which salt deposits are found. Sulfur, magnesium,
calcium, potassium, and trace minerals are all naturally
found alongside sodium chloride in the raw, unrefined form
of the salt that eventually—often, though not always, after
much industrial processing—ends up in (or on) our food.

I'll call unrefined, mineral-rich salt "true salt," since even
"sea salt" is a tricky phrase—because, like all other salt, it is
technically from the sea, so even if it is industrially refined
and stripped of its other minerals, it can still be labeled as "sea
salt." True salt is the unrefined salt mined from mineral-rich
deposits around the world, with its natural mineral content
left intact. Redmond's Real Salt, artisanal salts from small
operations across the world, Celtic sea salt, and Himalayan
salt all qualify.

The other minerals found in true salt interact with sodium chloride, and this interaction plays important roles in the
body. Potassium interacts with sodium chloride to modulate
the conveyance of nerve impulses and to enable muscles—
including the heart—to contract properly. ATP is required
for the carrying out of these functions, and magnesium is required for the synthesis of ATP. Calcium is moved from our
cells with the action of a sodium-calcium exchange protein.

Table salt, industrially processed so-called sea salt, and
even kosher salt are processed versions of the real thing,
with all naturally occurring minerals removed in the refining process. Interestingly, iodized salt, which is simply refined salt fortified with potassium iodide, a form of iodine,
wasn't created to compensate for iodine lost in the salt

refinement process. Iodine deficiency, a known cause of goiters, became more common in certain parts of the United States in the early 1900s due to iodine-poor soils and a lack of iodine-rich foods, like seafood. The government addressed this issue with the cheap, easy, shotgun approach of simply adding iodine to something everybody was already eating: salt. Iodized salt is in no way special; in fact, the iodization of salt may be connected to an increase in nongoiter thyroid disease. FDA labeling laws create the illusion that iodized salt is somehow better, as unrefined true salts that do not add iodine must state on their labels, "This salt does not contain iodide, a necessary nutrient." *Headsmack.*

Dietary salt first fell prey to mass industrialization in the 1800s. The novelty of the new science of food manufacturing made refined foods, in all their uniformity, alluring and desirable. It's the Starbucks syndrome: Wherever we go, we can get the same latte, with no surprises and no variation in taste or consistency. True salts weren't uniform enough, so refined salt became the order of the day.

True salt's unique mineral fingerprints and extra trace mineral nutrition were entirely erased by the refining industry. Thanks to some easy-pour, anticaking additives like dextrose and aluminum, this pure sodium chloride was totally uniform and conveniently packaged, and it still exists that way today. Morton Salt was among the first and the biggest salt-refining operations, and the salt-refining industry has only gotten bigger since the early 1900s. Morton is now a division of one of the world's largest salt-mining operations, which produces millions of tons of salt each year; some of that goes to road deicing, some to other industrial uses, and some to food. Processed food, that is.

And that's where it gets sadder than a chef without a spice rack.

Not only did the refining of salt strip away health-promoting trace minerals, but it also was a harbinger of things to come. While a pinch of even the most refined salt added to whole, nutritious food is no real problem—remember, our bodies need salt to survive—oversalted, undernutritious processed foods truly made a mess of things. The fascination with industrial food that prompted the refining of salt in the first place spiraled into the modern processed-food industry. This industry needs salt to survive.

Without excessive amounts of salt, according to journalist Michael Moss, cornflakes taste like metal, commercial ham products turn rubbery, processed cheese comes "unglued," bread made from refined grains becomes bitter, and nearly every processed food on the market takes on a totally intolerable taste. Salt's powerful, historically revered ability to reduce bitterness and enhance flavors has been harnessed to make nutritionally unconscionable, horrific-tasting profit products palatable.

And what else is in these processed foods? Refined sugars, processed grains, crop oils, and trans fats. Additives and synthetic preservatives. Artificial colors and flavors. A myriad of other ingredients that are far more devilish than salt has ever been. Salt is an innocent bystander that's been sucked into an industry that, for the last fifty years, has been making people incredibly sick. Most of the salt intake in the United States—nearly 75 percent—occurs through the vehicle of processed foods. Unfortunately, population studies on hypertension have confused the intake of salt with the intake of salt-laden processed foods.

The causal role of salt as an independent factor in chronic disease had little evidence to support it in the first place, but multiple policymakers still chose to throw the salt out with the seawater and recommend across-the-board sodium reduction for all individuals, not just the rare few with genetic salt sensitivities. In 1969, another shining example of nutrition hype becoming nutrition policy occurred on Senator George McGovern's watch as chairman of the Select Committee on Nutrition and Human Needs. Lewis Dahl, a physician who conducted several hypertension studies on rats, testified to the committee that excess salt caused hypertension, and because hypertension was associated with heart disease, he urged the committee not to wait for further research on salt but to press ahead with policy decisions that would end in the demonization of salt for its supposed role in heart disease. Despite inconclusive research in the following years that left Dahl's concerns anchored in ambiguity, salt paranoia set in. Across-the-board sodium reduction is ingrained (salt joke) in today's medical doctrine, though a 2011 letter published in the *British Medical Journal* called it "the largest delusion in the history of preventive medicine." Well said.

Hypertension and heart disease have nothing to do with the salt on our grass-fed steak. Or the steak itself, for that matter. Processed foods, not salt alone, are inseparable from the modern epidemics of hypertension and heart disease.

Hypertension is a term for chronically high blood pressure. Chronically high blood pressure stresses the arteries and, over time, can lead to arterial damage, heart attack, and stroke. Salt was pulled into the hypertensive fray because salt intake affects the fluid balance in the body, and when salt levels increase, a natural physiological cascade occurs wherein blood pressure temporarily rises to distribute excess salt in the appropriate amount of fluid in the body. Another physiological response to salt intake that helps our bodies balance salt concentration: thirst. Incidentally, that's why bars serve salty foods. It makes me—excuse me, bar patrons—drink more.

Here's the thing, though: Eating true salt on real foods, and the body's biological response to salt, doesn't equate to *chronically* high blood pressure; and a person with chronically high blood pressure isn't necessarily eating too much salt. However, over time, ingesting lots of processed foods— which have massive amounts of salt that we'd never eat in the form of pure salt alone—not only enables us to eat more salt than we need for proper function but also floods us with refined crop oils, trans fats, and refined sugars. It's no surprise, then, that chronically elevated *blood sugar* is strongly associated with high blood pressure, and this makes sense in light of the relationship among salt, sugar, and blood-sugar-spiking processed food.

Remember how I said that biologically, we can't live without salt? Though restricting processed food loaded with refined fats, sugars, and salt is good, restricting salt too much—as in not just avoiding processed food but eliminating that pinch of culinary, true salt on roasted vegetables or the finishing true salt on a steak—could be dangerous. One study showed that people who ate the lowest amounts of sodium died sooner than those who ate average amounts. Another study indicated that reduced sodium intake—*at levels recommended by the government*—might actually increase the risk of death from cardiovascular disease.

Perhaps salt's biological importance is the reason we have such a finely tuned taste for it. When our bodies need salt, it tastes amazing. When our bodies don't, it tastes like salivary glandular horror. The same amount of tasty salt in a homemade electrolyte drink that replenishes the body after a workout may be nearly unpalatable on a lazy day when the body's electrolyte stores haven't been depleted.

The culinary use of true salt in the preparation of real, natural foods, like meats, raw cheeses, and vegetables, is an everyday art. If salt is used to enhance, but not overpower, the taste of real food, it is nearly impossible to overuse from a nutritional standpoint. This is in stark contrast to the habitual overuse of hidden, refined salt in processed foods. As long as we eat only as much true, mineral-rich salt as tastes right to us, in a diet filled with real, whole foods, our salt intake should remain in perfect balance. As Mark Bitterman stated in *Salted: A Manifesto on the World's Most Essential Mineral,* "Eat all the salt you want, as long as you are the one doing the salting."

The right kind of salt—true salt—is naturally rich in other important minerals. This is part of what makes it special.

Our bodies need the "popular" minerals like calcium and sodium—the ones that get the most attention—but we need them in their natural state, not refined, alongside other nutrients that nature placed there for good reason. Throughout this book, the concept of nutrient synergy emerges again and again. It's inherent to real, natural foods, but it's not how conventional wisdom looks at what we eat. We're given recommended intakes for individual nutrients and are never told that the action of one nutrient also involves the actions of others.

Which minerals matter, and where are they found?

With the calcium and salt issues sorted out, there's still the matter of other minerals, what they mean to our bodies, how they work together, and where we can find them in food.

Calcium and salt are macrominerals. Macrominerals are the elements most abundant in the human body, and they include the electrolytes (or ions) that comprise our bodies' own electrical system. Macrominerals are calcium, sodium and chloride (which always occur together as salt), phosphorus, magnesium, potassium, and sulfur. With the exception of sulfur, all will function as electrolytes, although sodium chloride and potassium are the main electrolytes that control the critical balance of fluid inside and outside our cells.

Trace minerals are no less important, though they are needed in smaller amounts. This group includes iron, zinc, iodine, and selenium, among others. These minerals originate in the soil of the Earth or are dissolved in the water of the ocean, and they are absorbed by plants and algae, which concentrate them and pass them up the food chain through larger animals and sea creatures. Depleted soils produce depleted plants, and depleted plants mean poorly nourished creatures—yet another reason to opt for animals and plants raised as close to nature as possible, in nutrient-rich soils not stripped by conventional agriculture.

We're led to believe that the diet recommended by the government, which is largely centered around conventional agriculture, provides all we need, but not only is this false from the perspective of macronutrients—fat, carbohydrate, and protein—it's also false when it comes to minerals.

Though the most bioavailable minerals are found in creature foods, minerals and trace minerals are found in both plants and animals. However, modern grains, which are often plastered with health claims lauding their iron, zinc, and magnesium content, also carry the baggage of phytic acid, which you may remember from chapter 3. Phytic acid binds to minerals and prevents nutrients present in our food from being utilized by our bodies. This reduced bioavailability means that what we eat isn't always what we absorb. Think of it this way: Your pay stub says one number, but the actual bank deposit is half that. Not fair.

As we thumb through a few select critical minerals, bioavailability becomes a recurring theme. There's simply no mineral present in grains that we can't get in a more bioavailable form from animals, seafood, or a good dose of veggies. Sardines are rich in selenium and calcium; oysters are rich in zinc. Seafood, including sea vegetables, is rich in iodine. Green veggies grown in nutrient-rich soil are replete with magnesium. Red meats are rich in iron and zinc. Alongside those nutrients are the critical cofactors that enable the synergistic effects of real food.

Fun fact: The same minerals that are housed in certain bodily tissues in high concentrations are also *necessary* to the health of those same tissues. The most obvious example: Bones are made of calcium, magnesium, and phosphorus; and calcium, magnesium, and phosphorus are critical nutrients for bone health. This theme, and the theme of nutrient synergy, is repeated across the full spectrum of minerals.

Ready to wax nerdy on even more mineral minutiae? Let's start with phosphorus.

Phosphorus

This mineral is essential to every cell in the body, but it has suffered much the same fate as salt. It's often refined and added to processed foods in the form of phosphoric acid. Soft drinks and packaged junk foods are full of it, and, in that form, it can be dangerous; we take in too much, in unnatural proportions, and the consequences are tooth (calcium) erosion and bodily magnesium depletion. This is because, like calcium and magnesium, phosphorus is an important component of bone, and bone-supportive nutrition requires those three minerals to be in proper proportion to one another, as they occur in real food. Isolating them from one another—as processed foods do—creates a physiological imbalance that can erode teeth and deplete complementary nutrients in the body.

Phytic acid is actually the storage form of phosphorus. Beans, grains, and nuts contain phytic acid, and humans don't have the enzymes necessary to release all that phosphorus from storage; for that reason, less than half the phosphorus in these plants is actually liberated for use in our bodies. (Sidenote: Dibs on *Liberated Phosphorus* as a future band name.)

In its natural form, and when derived from the real food I won't shut up about, phosphorus occurs right alongside the nutrients we need to make use of it. Animal products—especially eggs, fish, homemade bone broth, and raw dairy—are sources of phosphorus and various phosphorus-cooperative nutrients, like vitamin D (which also works in concert with vitamin A), calcium, and magnesium.

Magnesium

Speaking of magnesium, it's a cofactor for vitamin D, potassium, and many other minerals, most notably calcium.

It keeps calcium in check in muscular function: Calcium is responsible for muscle contraction, and magnesium is responsible for muscle relaxation. Heart palpitations and muscle spasms may indicate low magnesium levels. More than half the magnesium in our bodies is concentrated in our bones and teeth; the rest in muscle and bodily fluid. It is found in high concentrations in the heart and brain.

Thanks to widespread deficiencies of magnesium in American soil, magnesium may be one of the most critically deficient minerals in our diet. Magnesium plays a vital role in everything from cellular energy production to enzymatic reactions to metabolic function, which means that deficiency promises a health smackdown of Hulk Hogan–esque proportions.

Plants use magnesium for the production of chlorophyll, which is necessary for photosynthesis; the greener the plant, the richer it is in magnesium. Dark, leafy greens grown in nutrient-dense soils are good sources of magnesium, and local farmer's markets are excellent resources for finding produce grown in healthy soils. Homemade bone broth, true sea salt, and raw milk also supply magnesium. Soaking in bathwater with Epsom salts, which are magnesium sulfate salts, lets us absorb both magnesium and sulfur through the skin. Sulfur is another critical mineral.

Sulfur

While magnesium, along with many other minerals, has long languished in the shadow of calcium, no mineral is as undervalued as sulfur. To date, there has been no government recommendation for daily sulfur intake, and although the government's endorsement isn't the most valuable voucher, this speaks to how neglected sulfur has been in the field of nutrition.

Perhaps this inattention is due to the fact that, for many years, sulfur was in abundant supply—so much so that, perhaps, we took it for granted. Animal proteins contain the sulfur amino acids. Egg yolks provide, and sunshine generates, forms of sulfur that, after decades of cholesterol and sunshine avoidance, are now in short supply. (Eat the yolks. Eat them.) While sauerkraut, leafy greens, garlic, and onions are good sources of sulfur, the deficiency of sulfur in nutrient-depleted soils may degrade sulfur content in the plants grown in them.

Sulfation, which is the addition of sulfate to nonsulfur molecules, is the critical process that sulfur deficiency can stonewall. We need sulfation in order to deploy the digestive substances that break down our food. Proper digestion is the body's means of extracting the bioavailable nutrition from food, so sulfur, through its digestive impact, actually interacts with the entire suite of nutrients we ingest. Sulfation is critical to the body's ability to detoxify noxious substances, like heavy metals, and is a component of the body's master antioxidant, glutathione.

Selenium

Antioxidants aren't exclusive to the foods that are famous for them. Too often we associate plants with antioxidant power, but blueberries, pomegranates, and açaï berries can't hold a candle to the antioxidant power of fat-soluble vitamins and minerals—including the mineral selenium, which is found in eggs (have I mentioned that it's important to *eat the yolks?*) as well as organ meats (be brave), muscle meats, and seafood. Brazil nuts are an excellent plant source of selenium, as they are grown in a region in Brazil with particularly selenium-rich soils.

Selenium, like sulfur, is a vital component of glutathione and plays a central role in protecting the body from free radical damage. Selenium also protects other antioxidants from damage and, in doing so, interacts with cofactors vitamins E and C.

Iodine

Selenium also interacts with iodine, which the thyroid depends on for building thyroid hormones. Iodized salt is not the only option for fortifying the diet with iodine, although it is a good solution for developing countries where seafood is not available and severe iodine deficiency is responsible for not just thyroid dysfunction but also severe developmental and cognitive disabilities in children. Raw milk from animals grazing on grass growing in iodine-rich soils is a good source of iodine, though pasteurized milk is low in iodine. All seafood, including fish, shellfish, and sea vegetables, is rich in iodine, but iodine from fish and shellfish carries the added benefit of being rich in—you guessed it—selenium. These cofactors exist alongside several other amazing nutrients, including taurine, vitamin D, cholesterol, and zinc.

Zinc

Zinc and selenium have another commonality. Sufficiency in these minerals means healthy swimmers (we should put that on a poster): They aid in the generation and protection of healthy sperm and sex hormones.

Zinc is important for both male and female reproductive health at all stages. It is critical for the formation of healthy gametes, as well as for overall hormonal health, and it continues to be important throughout pregnancy. As if that weren't enough, zinc also boosts the immune system, is essential to wound healing, and is crucial for eye health: It is concentrated in the retina, where it interacts with vitamin A to promote night vision.

Though nuts and seeds contain high levels of zinc, the best sources are creature foods: Red meat, shellfish, and other meats provide the most bioavailable zinc thanks to both the lack of phytic acid and the presence of sulfur-containing amino acids that improve zinc absorption. Unfortunately, these foods don't often make "best sources" lists thanks to the nutrition dogma that surrounds them—ironic, since conventional-wisdom-friendly whole grains, often touted for their zinc content, actually contain phytic acid that cripples zinc utilization, so much so that strict vegetarians may need as much as 50 percent more zinc than meat-eaters to achieve the same rate of zinc absorption.

Iron

Our final mineral for the day, iron, shares several characteristics with zinc. As with zinc, our ability to absorb iron depends on the source. Plant-based iron is known as *nonheme,* and although animal products also contain nonheme iron, they contain the easily absorbed form of iron called *heme iron* as well. Iron in plant sources, like grains and legumes, suffers from the same fate as other minerals: It's bound up in phytic acid, which can reduce absorption to a pathetic 2 percent.

Iron is likely the best-known mineral, and it's not one to shortchange—and not just because severe iron deficiency can cause taste buds to lose sensation, which means that we can't taste our crab-topped filet. Heme is a component of hemoglobin, which transports oxygen throughout the body. Iron deficiency anemia causes reduced delivery of oxygen to bodily tissue. Like zinc, iron is vital to immune and reproductive function, and deficiency can cause low birth weight.

Though I could go on about minerals forever—that's just the kind of boring, overobsessed nutrition freak I am—we can only truly touch the tip of the iceberg. Minerals interact with other nutrients, and one another, in the most intricate ways, many of which science doesn't fully understand yet. Further, while many of these minerals are vital to our long-term health, that doesn't mean we need to flood our bodies with them. *Trace minerals* are needed in small quantities, so there's no need to gorge on Brazil nuts or eat a juicy steak at every meal. A little goes a long way.

Most important, we absolutely cannot obsess over individual nutrient allowances to the tune of supplements, because supplements can't possibly contain the suite of remarkable cofactors inherent in real food.

So what to do?

....

In a nutshell: Go full-on food badass. Eat what your ancestors ate.

Unfortunately, the various so-called "healthy diets" that are mainstream favorites are simply not dense in nutrition. A standard low-fat diet based on lean white meat over salad greens and the occasional veggie burger won't cut it—it's missing all the critical nutrition found in natural fats. Plant-based diets fall short as well: Many vital nutrients are more bioavailable from creature foods, and some are found only in creature foods. And a standard junk food diet—whether based on true junk food or prepackaged diet junk food—certainly doesn't provide the nutrition we need.

The foods of our ancestors are truly the missing link when it comes to making sure we get all the nutrients we need from real food. We've been led to believe that we need vitamin pills and supplements as "insurance" for wherever our diet might fall short—but what we actually need are all the fun, weird, badass foods that, up to just a few decades ago, were common, even in our grandparents' diet. These are the foods that provide all the nutrition we need. They're modern-day sources of old-school nutrition. And they are healthy as hell.

I'm talking about organ meats like liver from properly raised animals, which is perhaps the best possible source of B vitamins, folate, and trace minerals. I'm talking about cod liver oil, which is rich in vitamins A and D, and butter and raw milk from grass-fed cows, which are rich in vitamin K_2.

I'm talking about egg yolks, dammit, which are among the most nutrient-rich powerhouses on the planet, loaded with vitamin A, vitamin D, choline, sulfur, selenium, and healthy cholesterol. I'm talking about seafood, like sardines and oysters, which contain zinc, taurine, and iodine. I'm talking about bone marrow, which is about as caveman as it gets, but which is also found in culinary beauties like osso buco (if you're fancy).

I'm also talking about bone broth, also called stock. (In the culinary world, there are a few minor differences between the two that affect flavor but not nutrition.) Whatever you call it, it is the savory, healing, nutrient-filled liquid made by boiling bones, usually along with vegetables; this practice has a long history in cultures across the globe. Bone broth—whether it's made from poultry, beef, or fish—is the ultimate in thoughtful, grateful, no-waste, budget-conscious cooking; even the bones of nutritious animals are used once the meat has been enjoyed.

Unfortunately, we've ruined the traditional stuff with pathetic imitations found in cartons and cans or dehydrated into bouillon, but the truth is, there's no substitute for the real thing, because traditional bone broths are as rich in minerals as the bones they're made from. Bones are reservoirs of calcium, magnesium, and potassium, and the matrix of connective tissue that dissolves into bone broth is also rich in skin-loving, healing nutrients, such as glycine and gelatin—it's basically a face-lift in a cup. Adding mineral-rich, unrefined true salt means even greater flavor and nutrition for every sauce, gravy, soup, and stew it's added to. And all we've got to do is boil some bones.

Many of these nutrient-filled, nose-to-tail goodies are actually available in modern restaurants—they cost a full arm, of course, at trendy eateries, yet they were budget-conscious staples in old-school kitchens. The nutrient value per calorie alone is enough to make them worth learning to appreciate. And the street cred you'll earn makes becoming an odd-bits aficionado that much more fun.

Remember, *none of these foods are weird.* They're just foods many of us weren't brought up on, in that era of low-fat fears and cholesterol paranoia, when anything out of a package was in vogue. These are foods we're not used to. They've fallen out of memory in modern America, but in many parts of the world, they're still dinnertime staples. Let's bring 'em back.

All told, eating nose-to-tail doesn't mean that your food has to seem strange. A typical day could start with eggs and smoked salmon alongside a roasted sweet potato topped with grass-fed butter and a dab of roasted bone marrow. Right there you have vitamins A, D, and K_2, omega-3, and healthy fat, protein, and carbs. Lunch, eaten outside under the afternoon sun for some vitamin D, could be smoky paprika chicken thighs over greens with homemade bacon-mustard vinaigrette—vitamins and minerals galore. Add a side of sulfur-rich sauerkraut, which has the added benefit of being rich in probiotics, for bonus points. Dinner: No-bean chili made with homemade broth and "hidden" liver. That's zinc, iron, minerals, healthy complete protein, and more.

Just eat and enjoy. Don't count nutrients. Don't worry about how much you're getting, because with real food, you're getting plenty. So the strategy is simple: Eat real food. Find a decent recipe for liver pâté, preferably in a cookbook with *Paleo* in the title, and buy healthy, whole ingredients. You're set.

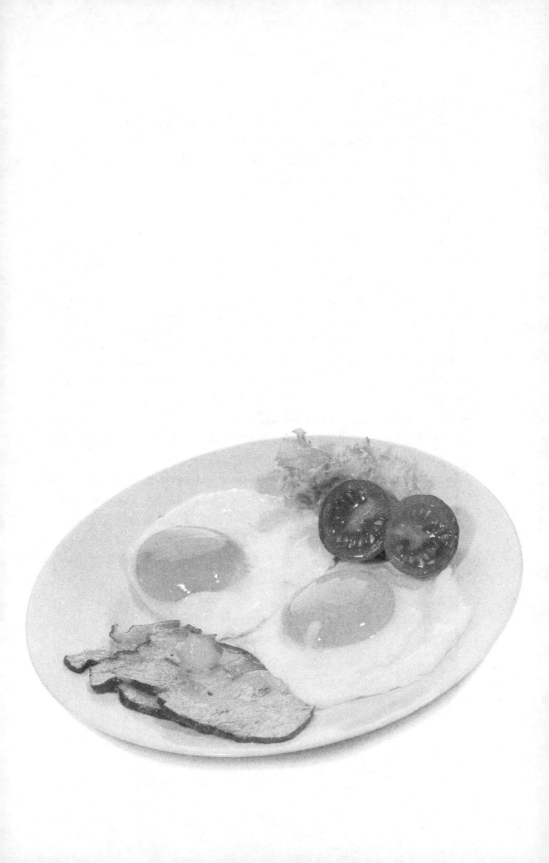

conclusion

Where we've been

My Paleo journey began with the basics. I eliminated the junk, focused on real food as best I could, and continued to learn both the how and the why, step by step and little by little. The easy part was eating real food. The hardest part was realizing that I'd believed so many lies about the foods I ate every single day, and that those lies had, for years, driven my deranged relationship with food.

Some of those lies took root long ago and grew out of ignorance. When trans fats entered the food supply in the early 1900s, for example, it wasn't part of some conspiracy intended to destroy our health at the cellular level. At the time, the technology seemed promising: It could make foods last longer. The potential consequences of fundamentally altering the molecular structure of a food weren't even on the food industry radar. Yet by the time heart disease was recognized as a full-blown epidemic in the 1960s, there were many who considered trans fats a suspect. By that time, however, the crop oil industry had built a profitable business around "vegetable" oils and the trans fats made from them. And our nation's health continued to decline.

From there, lies were perpetuated by industries with much to gain from keeping their own products profitable. Cautions about trans fats were ignored and even forced out of official government policy. Misplaced fears over the unproven dangers of cholesterol and saturated fat quickly became ammunition for the marketing schemes of the crop oil industry, whose by-products helped support the confining and improper feeding of animals raised for food. Concerned activists fight the factory farm but often don't realize how intertwined it is with the so-called health foods made from industrial crops that line every aisle of every grocery store in the nation.

In the course of just over a century, we've tossed away real, nourishing foods, often in favor of factory-made industrial products that somehow claim to be better than the real thing.

At first, it's hard to believe the extent of nutrition misinformation that has been spread, institutionalized, and commercialized for decades. It seems impossible. Yet to look around at the ill, the unhappy, the confused—it's not only possible, it's true.

And we're suffering for it. The diseases we were supposed to fight with the dietary changes of conventional wisdom are on the rise. Heart disease and stroke, obesity, hypertension, and depression are a constant challenge to public health, despite our efforts to do the right thing. Diet books are continual best sellers, and almost no one is satisfied with their health. We're living the lies.

Fighting the lies means learning the truth: the truth about nutrients, food history, and how we got to a place where we considered a breakfast of boxed cardboard topped with skim milk a better choice than a breakfast of whole eggs, grass-fed steak, sweet potatoes, and greens.

Fighting the lies also means realizing that our own perceived failures and frustrations aren't due to our "bad genes" or lack of willpower. We all do the best we can. Even the truly gross stuff we do in the name of better health (like eat flavorless cardboardlike fiber cereal drenched in soy milk) is consumed with good (though perhaps delusional) intentions. The problem is not that we're really bad at taking good advice. It's that we've been *really good* at taking *horrible* advice.

That horrible advice has come in many forms—there's no one thing to demonize. Multiple things can cause us harm: Conventional wisdom. Diet dogma. Processed food. Processed food disguised as healthy food. An overabundance of crappy carbs. Damaged, processed fats. Nutrient-stripped soil and nutrient-poor food.

Fear of real food, however, is the most damaging demon of all. It's what inspired this whole lie-fighting book.

Where we're going

The Paleo community—and, if you've made it this far, you are a welcome part of that community—is doing something unprecedented. We are crushing nutritional dogma. We are fighting the lies we've been fed for years, and our health is better for it. We are bringing the way we eat back into harmony with how our bodies work.

What we're doing goes deeper than dieting. We are reclaiming our health. (Fist pump.)

Our choices stretch beyond what we're doing for our own bodies: We are educated eaters, demanding more from our food system. There is a way to produce food that does not involve factory farming or industrial agriculture, and the foods produced outside those systems are the ones that truly nourish our bodies.

We are activists simply by virtue of our choices. Every meal we eat that's free of processed junk, crop oils, and refined industrial ingredients is a major statement. It's a vote against the status quo.

We're flipping conventional wisdom the bird. And man, does it feel good.

Eating cholesterol-rich animal foods and fat from natural sources—like properly raised animals, seafood, whole plants, and unrefined oils—is pretty dang revolutionary given the last half-century of cholesterol paranoia and anti-fat indoctrination. It also means a diet pretty dang rich in fat-soluble vitamins and the raw materials the body deeply needs for cellular and hormonal health. For decades, people of all ages—kids and adults alike—have been starved of these foundational nutrients. We're changing that.

Eating whole-creature protein is not just a way to get all the amino acids we need in the right proportions. It's an act of defiance against the many myths we've believed about how food is raised and where we belong in the food chain. Factory farming is not the only way to get meat to the masses. Small, sustainable farms and homesteads are emerging everywhere to supply products from properly raised animals to their communities. The more we ask for food produced in this manner, the more that need will be met. We're doing that.

Eating vegetables and fruits instead of conventional grains, "whole" or otherwise, may not sound radical, but it truly is. Industrial agriculture, the originator of most modern grain-based foods, has tentacles that creep into almost everything we're fighting against: Factory farming. Soil degradation. Highly processed oils. Refined foods stripped of nutrition. A life of confusion about what we should eat and why. We're fixing that.

Eating nose-to-tail and enjoying the often-forgotten, nutrient-rich foods that our ancestors ate means pulling as much nutrition as possible from the animals we consume. It's an incredible way to show appreciation for the food we're so fortunate to have available to us. We can (when we're ready) begin to demonstrate that.

To become a nutrient-seeker rather than a calorie-counter is to become deeply connected with your food and your body. It is transformational.

How we get there

....

Where this transformation takes you is entirely up to you. Humans are adaptable, and there is no one diet that's right for everyone. There *are*, however, guidelines that work for everyone:

- Processed crap isn't good. Whether we're talking crop oils, low-fat processed foods, so-called health foods with a long list of unpronounceable ingredients, or crop-based carbohydrates processed into packaged cereal, pasta, and bread, the processed stuff is a profit-first, health-last proposition. The companies that make them have lied to us and tried their darnedest to hide the truth. Not cool.

- Whole foods with a long history in the human diet will provide the body with incredibly dense nutrition. Most important, properly raised animal products and seafood have been a part of healthy humans' diets for thousands of years. Don't avoid them for fear of fat and cholesterol. They're not the enemy. They're some of the best friends we could hope for.

- Nutrients and knowledge are good. Knowing where the nutrients are is what turns a dieter into a smart eater. Nutrients come with the food of our ancestors, and they also come from responsible sun exposure.

- Food quality is important. Factory food, whether derived from plants or animals, doesn't provide adequate nutrition. Plants grown in well-managed soil, as well as properly raised animals, provide the best nutrition possible.

From there, it's all about you.

Want animal protein at every meal? If it works for you, more power to you. Prefer to base your meals around healthy veggies, with animal products playing a supporting role?

Follow your instincts. High-fat? Go for it. High-carb? That's cool *if it works for you.* Yes, I think animal products are important. But one person's daily steak-'n'-eggs may be another person's weekly oyster stew. There is no one-size-fits-all prescription for how much to eat of what and when, and anyone who says there is has something questionable to sell. We all need to decide how to eat based on what works best for us. And knowing the truth about food makes it easy, exciting, and fun to make choices that improve and sustain our health.

It's all about information. Learning the history of food, where the nutrients are, and what works for *you* is far more effective in the long term than using Paleo as a straitjacket that limits your choices. Paleo should simply be a framework for making better choices. Remember how I said that this book is about learning from our ancestors and adopting the modern versions of the behaviors that kept them healthy? That means context is important. We're not replaying some distant history bite by bite; we're learning from our ancestors, seeking nutrients, and busting myths. It's not as complex as it sounds. You've already read umpteen pages about it. Heck, you're practically an expert at this point. It's about the lessons of good science, history, anthropology, and biology. It's about being in tune with who we are and what we need—no packaging, processing, diet books, or lists of arbitrary rules required.

This book was written to communicate a few simple ideas: Real, unprocessed foods—including animal products—are the fuel that makes us awesome, and there's no substitute in a box, bag, or capsule. We don't have to fear real food. We can outsmart the status quo. None of that is baggage or burdensome. It's tasty, it's rebellious, and it's fun.

Where to begin

....

I advocate real food, from sources that raise, grow, or catch it right. That's it. Even so, this isn't an all-or-nothing manifesto. Start where you can, when you can, and do the best you can. Just start—because the world of supermarket jargon is only getting more confusing, the world of industrial pesticides more poisonous, and the problem of soil depletion more insidious. The important thing is that you start, and once you start, keep on going.

Local farmers and growers who take care of the soil with as much dedication as they show to their animals and plants are producing the most nutritious foods. So the best we can do is to try to buy local foods from trusted sources. If you can, talk to the people who raise, grow, or supply your food. Ask questions about how they manage pests, pastures, and the health of the soil. Learn from them, and thank them by becoming their customer. Better yet, grow your own food if you can, and if you already do, start teaching others to do the same.

Of course, we can't all have grass-fed beef and wild-caught fish and locally grown sweet potatoes for every meal. That's *fine*. (Although if you can, and you want to start by making sweeping changes to every meal and every item in your kitchen, rock on with your real-food self.) When my husband and I decided that we wanted to buy some of our food from local farms rather than the big-box grocery store, we took it slow. We squirreled away spare change for monthly trips to the farmer's market to fill a small bag. We shifted our expenses where we could, slowly cutting back on things like gourmet coffee and premium cable. We made sure to turn off the lights when we left the house and wore our jeans a few more times before we washed them. As much as possible, we used every part of the animals we ate, including making nutrient-rich broth from the bones. We tried (and mostly failed) to grow our own food. Little steps or big steps. It's up to you.

It has never been easier to take this leap. Resources, recipes, and lifestyle advice are as close as the Internet. Farmer's markets, local farmers, community-supported agriculture, and even free gardening lessons are cropping up in cities across the world, and it's all connected by the web. A few years back, it was nearly impossible to find a local farmer's market, let alone a whole database of nationwide resources for great, local food. Now, all it takes is an Internet connection—or, if you're old school, a local library. (And if you're so inclined, head over to EatTheYolks.com for my free online resource guide.)

Feel as if you don't have time to make changes? I promise, you do—because you don't have to make all the changes all at once. You can make them one by one, as you're comfortable. If you ever go to the grocery store, you have a moment to read—and be horrified by—the ingredients labels on the food they sell. If you watch any amount of TV, you have time to try cooking something new. If you spend a nanosecond on Facebook, you have time to Google a few things, like your growing region or the address of your local farmer's market.

Just because you can't be fully invested *now* doesn't mean that you can't take small steps toward a more informed, more nutritious way of eating. Though the greatest benefits may come once you're fully engaged, your path to getting there is yours and yours alone.

I won't pretend that all processed foods or common so-called health foods, or even properly prepared grains, beans, oats, and other staples of the health food section, will destroy your body, quash your dreams, or tell your kids there's no Santa Claus. They probably won't. But can they do all the amazing things that the food we've talked about in this book can do? Probably not. Still, the choices are yours, and only yours. Remember this: You are not dieting. You are living.

You are the boss of you. If there's any overarching problem with how we interact with our food, from what we choose to eat to why we choose to eat it, it's that we let somebody else—government, guru, or book writer—make the rules for us.

Just make sure you have all the information. Live by your own rules, but build those rules on a firm foundation. With this book, I've tried to provide the facts behind our most common food myths, and I hope that you'll continue to question the latest studies and nutrition recommendations. Remember: Knowing is half the battle.

Someone once told me that if it's worth doing, it's worth doing poorly at first. So go out there and royally suck at finding, growing, or cooking healthy food. I'll be right there with you, every step of the way.

You are worthy of the truth, and you're worthy of good nutrition.

nutrition in 100 words

Seek real, nutrient-filled food, as close to its natural state as possible: whole, unprocessed, unmodified, and unrefined.

Pretend the modern supermarket doesn't exist. Choose foods that could be hunted or gathered—food that has *always* been food.

Support local, responsible producers.

Eat vegetables and fruits. Eat meat and fat from properly raised animals, eggs, and seafood. Enjoy cold-pressed oils and plants rich in healthy fats, like coconut, avocado, and olives.

Drink water.

Incorporate superfoods: fermented vegetables and beverages, homemade bone broth, and organ meats (if you dare).

Above all, ditch obsessive behavior and "diets."

Question conventional wisdom.

Eat real food.

acknowledgments

This book changed me. Writing it was an education. I began writing with the belief that I knew what I wanted to say; many months, many tears, and many proud moments later, I realize that this book took on a life of its own. It is more than I knew I could say, more than I ever thought I'd be able to put in one place. I know more now than I knew when I began this journey, and at the same time, I feel as if I know less. There is more information out there, more ideas, more knowledge and inspiration about food and health than could ever be gathered in one place. I've done my best, and I will never stop seeking.

So much gratitude goes to my husband, Spence, my greatest love and best friend, a man of extraordinary integrity and talent who makes me smile and laugh every day, and who drives me crazy in the best possible way. You have been *everything* to this process. I love you, I respect you, I am forever changed because of you.

To my parents: You are the people I respect most in this world, the people who gave me my sense of humor and, of course, my addiction to (and ability to quote) classic television and cinema. Dad, it's your example that helped me understand what it means to have integrity; Mom, it's your sense of purpose and perseverance—and your beautiful poetry—that inspired me throughout this writing process. My greatest hope is to make you both proud!

To my sister: You are a bright, shining light. You are hilarious. *We* are hilarious. I've never laughed so hard at nothing as I have with you. It's good for my soul! I've never been more fiercely proud of, or so deeply inspired by, anyone. Your beauty, depth, humor, and capabilities astound me. You are my closest friend and I'm so grateful for you.

To my grandmother: You are the most perceptive, well-read, intelligent woman I know. You embody true wisdom and principle.

To Mary, John, Sarah, Greg, Amy, and RayLynn: Thank you for being supportive, unconditional, and for providing a solid foundation. I am blessed to have all of you in my life.

To my military friends: Thank you for being a warm, welcoming second family, and thank you for your service and sacrifice.

To Diane, my podcast partner, colleague, and partner in travel-related hijinks: Thank you for believing in me. Thank you for being a force in the community, a constant source of inspiration, and an honest and true friend.

To Bill and Hayley, who are the reason I got to write this book: Thank you. You'll never know the extent of my respect for you both, and my gratitude for our friendship.

To my Steve's Club family; my friends (I consider you family) Quinn, Jessie, Christie, Layna, and Sally; and to Coach Rut, who started it all: You have been endless sources of inspiration to me. Thank you.

To those who have read my blog, listened to the Balanced Bites podcasts, and attended my workshops; and to the many amazing people I've met thanks to those endeavors: Your support is the reason I've been able to turn my passion into my profession. It is because of you, and all I've learned from you, that I was able to write this book. This is an incredible gift. Thank you.

To the Price-Pottenger Nutrition Foundation, the Nutritional Therapy Association, and the Farm to Consumer Legal Defense Fund: Thank you for introducing me to the work of Weston A. Price, which is preserved through the tireless work of the Weston A. Price Foundation, and for being so utterly dedicated to the cause of making real food, properly raised animals, and nutrition truths available to all. Immense gratitude also goes to Chris Masterjohn, Denise Minger, Mary Enig, and Fred Kummerow for being brave truth-tellers, and for analyzing and distilling volumes of scientific information for those of us who want to spread the word.

To Erin: Your hard work gave me clarity, and this book would be nothing but a long string of blather without you. I'm truly sorry for what you had to go through, but so grateful to have had you soldiering away to make this happen. I'll never be able to thank you enough.

And finally, to Erich: Thank you for your enthusiasm, for your dedication, and, most of all, for this opportunity. It is, quite literally, a dream come true.

sources

INTRODUCTION

Carbohydrates in Human Nutrition. Rome: Food and Agriculture Organization of the United Nations, 1997. FAO Food and Nutrition Paper. FAO Corporate Document Repository. www.fao.org/docrep/W8079E/w8079e00.htm

Fiscal Year 2012 Annual Report. Academy of Nutrition and Dietetics. www.eatright.org/Media/content.aspx?id=5202#.UoKxwpRAQ0h

Freedman, David H. "Lies, Damned Lies, and Medical Science." *The Atlantic* (November 2010): n.p. 4 Oct. 2010. www.theatlantic.com/magazine/archive/2010/11/lies-damned-lies-and-medical-science/308269/

Hite, Adele H., et al. "In the Face of Contradictory Evidence: Report of the Dietary Guidelines for Americans Committee." *Nutrition* 26, no. 10 (2010): 915–24. www.nutritionjrnl.com/article/S0899-9007(10)00289-3/fulltext

Ioannidis, John P. A. "Why Most Published Research Findings Are False." *PLOS Medicine* 2, no. 8 (2005): E124. www.plosmedicine.org/article/info:doi/10.1371/journal.pmed.0020124

Price, Weston A. *Nutrition and Physical Degeneration: A Comparison of Primitive and Modern Diets and Their Effects*, 8th ed. La Mesa, Calif.: Price-Pottenger Nutrition Foundation, 2008.

CHAPTER 1: FAT

Bonthuis, M., M. C. B. Hugues, T. I. Ibiebele, et al. "Dairy Consumption and Patterns of Mortality of Australian Adults." *European Journal of Clinical Nutrition* 64, no. 6 (2010): 569–77.

Campbell-McBride, Natasha. *Put Your Heart in Your Mouth*. Cambridge, U.K.: Medinform, 2007.

Chow, Ching Kuang. *Fatty Acids in Foods and Their Health Implications*. New York: Marcel Dekker, 1992.

Colpo, Anthony. *The Great Cholesterol Con: Why Everything You've Been Told About Cholesterol, Diet and Heart Disease Is Wrong!* Raleigh, N.C.: Lulu, 2006.

Dayspring, Thomas, and James A. Underberg. "A Preventable Soprano Death." *LecturePad.org*, n.d. www.lecturepad.org/index.php/commentaries-and-opinions/1148-a-preventable-soprano-death

Dona, Artemis, and Ioannis Arvanitoyannis. "Health Risks of Genetically Modified Foods." *Critical Reviews in Food Science and Nutrition* 49, no. 2 (2009): 164–75.

Enig, Mary G. *Know Your Fats: The Complete Primer for Understanding the Nutrition of Fats, Oils, and Cholesterol.* Silver Spring, Md.: Bethesda Press, 2000.

Enig, Mary G., and Sally Fallon. "The Oiling of America." Weston A. Price Foundation (2000). www.westonaprice.org/knowyourfats/oiling.html

Erasmus, Udo. *Fats That Heal, Fats That Kill: The Complete Guide to Fats, Oils, Cholesterol, and Human Health.* Burnaby, B.C., Canada: Alive, 1993.

Graveline, Duane. *Lipitor, Thief of Memory: Statin Drugs and the Misguided War on Cholesterol.* Haverford, Pa.: Infinity, 2004.

Hauter, Wenonah. *Foodopoly: The Battle Over the Future of Food and Farming in America.* New York: New Press, 2012.

Hu, Frank B., JoAnn E. Manson, and Walter C. Willett. "Types of Dietary Fat and Risk of Coronary Heart Disease: A Critical Review." *Journal of the American College of Nutrition* 20, no. 1 (2001): 5–19. http://jacn.manchester-mcmexpo.net/content/20/1/5.full

Institute of Shortening and Edible Oils. www.iseo.org

Jolly, David. "Hoping to Save Bees, Europe to Vote on Pesticide Ban." *New York Times* (March 14, 2013). www.nytimes.com/2013/03/15/business/global/hoping-to-save-bees-europe-to-vote-on-pesticide-ban.html

Kelly, Margie. "Top 7 Genetically Modified Crops." *The Huffington Post* (October 30, 2012). www.huffingtonpost.com/margie-kelly/genetically-modified-food_b_2039455.html

Konstantinov, Igor E., Nicolai Mejevoi, and Nikolai M. Anchikov. "Nikolai N. Anchikov and His Theory of Atherosclerosis." *Texas Heart Institute Journal* 33, no. 4 (2006): 417–23. PubMed Central. www.ncbi.nlm.nih.gov/pmc/articles/PMC1764970/

Liu, KeShun. *Soybeans: Chemistry, Technology, and Utilization.* New York: Chapman & Hall, 1997.

Mann, George. Foreword. *In Fat: It's Not What You Think,* by Connie Leas. New York: Prometheus Books, 2008.

Masterjohn, Chris. "Learning, Your Memory, and Cholesterol." *Cholesterol-and-health.com* (July 2005). www.cholesterol-and-health.com/Memory-And-Cholesterol.html

———. "High Cholesterol and Heart Disease—Myth or Truth?" *Cholesterol-and-health.com* (August 23, 2008). www.cholesterol-and-health.com/Does-Cholesterol-Cause-Heart-Disease-Myth.html

————. "How Essential Are the Essential Fatty Acids? The PUFA Report Part 1: A Critical Review of the Requirement for Polyunsaturated Fatty Acids." *Cholesterol-and-health.com Special Reports* 1, no. 2 (2008). www.cholesterol-and-health.com/PUFA-Special-Report.html

————. "Precious Yet Perilous." *Wise Traditions in Food, Farming, and the Healing Arts* (Fall 2010). Weston A. Price Foundation. www.westonaprice.org/know-your-fats/precious-yet-perilous

————. "Good Fats, Bad Fats: Separating Fact from Fiction." *Wise Traditions in Food, Farming, and the Healing Arts* (Spring 2012). Weston A. Price Foundation. www.westonaprice.org/know-your-fats/good-fats-bad-fats-separating-fact-from-fiction

Mayo Clinic. "Trans Fat Is Double Trouble for Your Heart Health" (May 6, 2011). www.mayoclinic.com/health/trans-fat/CL00032

Planck, Nina. *Real Food: What to Eat and Why*. New York: Bloomsbury USA, 2006.

Price, Weston A. *Nutrition and Physical Degeneration: A Comparison of Primitive and Modern Diets and Their Effects*, 8th ed. La Mesa, Calif.: Price-Pottenger Nutrition Foundation, 2008.

Shaw, Judith. *Trans Fats: The Hidden Killer in Our Food*. New York: Pocket Books, 2004.

Siri-Tarino, Patty W., Qi Sun, Frank B. Hu, and Ronald M. Krauss. "Meta-analysis of Prospective Cohort Studies Evaluating the Association of Saturated Fat with Cardiovascular Disease." *American Journal of Clinical Nutrition* 91, no. 3 (2010): 535–46. http://ajcn.nutrition.org/content/91/3/535.full.pdf+html?sid=892a56ce-29fb-444c-b903-b97356952587

Stehbens, W. E. "Anitschkow and the Cholesterol Over-Fed Rabbit." *Cardiovascular Pathology* 8, no. 3 (1999): 177–78.

Stuijvenberg, Johannes Hermanus van. Margarine: *An Economic, Social and Scientific History*, 1869–1969. Liverpool: Liverpool University Press, 1969.

United States Senate, Select Committee on Nutrition and Human Needs. "Dietary Goals for the United States, Supplemental Views." Washington, D.C.: U.S. Government Printing Office, 1977. Hathi Trust Digital Library. http://babel.hathitrust.org/cgi/pt?id=umn.31951d00283417h;view=1up;seq=146

Watts, G., et al. "Effects on Coronary Artery Disease of Lipid-Lowering Diet, or Diet Plus Cholestyramine, in the St. Thomas' Atherosclerosis Regression Study (STARS)." *The Lancet* 339, no. 8793 (1992): 563–69.

CHAPTER 2: PROTEIN

Appleton, B. Scott, and T. Colin Campbell. "Inhibition of Aflatoxin-Initiated Preneoplastic Liver Lesions by Low Dietary Protein." *Nutrition and Cancer* 3, no. 4 (1982): 200–206.

Aro, Antti, et al. "Inverse Association Between Dietary and Serum Conjugated Linoleic Acid and Risk of Breast Cancer in Postmenopausal Women." *Nutrition and Cancer* 38, no. 2 (2000): 151–57.

Blum, Miriam, Mordechai Averbuch, Yoram Wolman, and Alexander Aviram. "Protein Intake and Kidney Function in Humans: Its Effect on 'Normal Aging.'" *JAMA Internal Medicine* 149, no. 1 (1989): 211–12.

Brosnan, John T., and Margaret E. Brosnan. "The Sulfur-Containing Amino Acids: An Overview." *Journal of Nutrition* 136, no. 6 (2006): 1636S–1640S.

Campbell, T. Colin, and Thomas M. Campbell II. *The China Study: The Most Comprehensive Study of Nutrition Ever Conducted and the Startling Implications for Diet, Weight Loss, and Long-Term Health.* Dallas: BenBella Books, 2005.

Chamovitz, Daniel. *What a Plant Knows: A Field Guide to the Senses.* New York: Farrar, Straus and Giroux, 2012. Kindle edition.

Champeau, Rachel. "Most Heart Attack Patients' Cholesterol Levels Did Not Indicate Cardiac Risk." *UCLA Newsroom* (January 11, 2009). http://newsroom.ucla.edu/portal/ucla/majority-of-hospitalized-heart-75668.aspx

Chen, Junshi. *Diet, Life-Style, and Mortality in China: A Study of the Characteristics of 65 Chinese Counties.* Oxford, U.K.: Oxford University Press, 1990.

Clark, Richard M., Lili Yao, Li She, and Harold C. Furr. "A Comparison of Lycopene and Astaxanthin Absorption from Corn Oil and Olive Oil Emulsions." *Lipids* 35, no. 7 (2000): 803–806.

Cordain, Loren, and T. Colin Campbell. "The Protein Debate." *Catalyst Athletics* (March 19, 2008). www.catalystathletics.com/articles/article.php?articleID=50

Cousens, Gabriel. "The Elusive B12." Blog post. *Dr. Cousens' Blog.* Dr. Cousens' Tree of Life Rejuvenation Center (March 18, 2011). www.gabriel-cousens.com/DRCOUSENS/DRCOUSENSBLOG/tabid/364/language/en-US/~/Default.aspx?PostID=149&tabid=364&language=en-US

Ellison, Shane. *Hidden Truth about Cholesterol-Lowering Drugs: How to Avoid Heart Disease Naturally,* rev. ed. Northglenn, Colo.: Health Myths Publishing, 2006.

Enig, Mary G., and Sally Fallon. "The Oiling of America." Weston A. Price Foundation (2000). www.westonaprice.org/know-your-fats/the-oiling-of-america

Fairlie, Simon. *Meat: A Benign Extravagance.* White River Junction, Vt.: Chelsea Green Publishing, 2010.

Fallon, Sally, Mary G. Enig, Kim Murray, and Marion Dearth. *Nourishing Traditions: The Cookbook That Challenges Politically Correct Nutrition and the Diet Dictocrats.* Washington, D.C.: NewTrends Publishing, 2001.

Felton, C. V., et al. "Dietary Polyunsaturated Fatty Acids and Composition of Human Aortic Plaques." *The Lancet* 344, no. 8931 (1994): 1195–96.

"Finding Aid for John Harvey Kellogg Papers, 1869–1965." Michigan Historical Collections, Bentley Historical Library, University of Michigan. http://quod. lib.umich.edu/b/bhlead/umich-bhl-89500?rgn=main;view=text

Food, Inc. Robert Kenner, director. Movie One, 2008. Film.

Golomb, Beatrice A. "Cholesterol and Violence: Is There a Connection?" *Annals of Internal Medicine* 128, no. 6 (1998): 478–87.

Heaney, Robert P. "Protein Intake and Bone Health: The Influence of Belief Systems on the Conduct of Nutritional Science." *American Journal of Clinical Nutrition* 73, no. 1 (2001): 5–6. http://ajcn.nutrition.org/content/73/1/5.full?ijk ey=4cb6e2c476005c7b83fa6ad532f803db8a3b65ec&keytype2=tf_ipsecsha

Herbert, Victor. "Vitamin B-12: Plant Sources, Requirements, and Assay." *American Journal of Clinical Nutrition* 48, no. 3 (1988): 852–58. http://ajcn. nutrition.org/content/48/3/852.full.pdf

Iacobbo, Karen, and Michael Iacobbo. *Vegetarian America: A History.* Westport, Conn.: Praeger, 2004.

International Programme on Chemical Safety. Environmental Health Criteria. *Ammonia (EHC 54)* (1986). www.inchem.org/documents/ehc/ehc/ehc54. htm

Jackson, Alan A., Chandarika Persaud, Tracey S. Meakins, and Rafe Bundy. "Urinary Excretions of 5-L-Oxoproline (Pyroglutamic Acid) Is Increased in Normal Adults Consuming Vegetarian or Low Protein Diets." *Journal of Nutrition* 126, no. 11 (1996): 2813–22. http://jn.nutrition.org/ content/126/11/2813.full.pdf+html

Jones, Peter J. H. "Dietary Cholesterol Feeding Suppresses Human Cholesterol Synthesis Measured by Deuterium Incorporation and Urinary Mevalonic Acid Levels." *Arteriosclerosis, Thrombosis, and Vascular Biology* 16 (1996): 1222–28. http://atvb.ahajournals.org/content/16/10/1222.long

Keith, Lierre. *The Vegetarian Myth: Food, Justice, and Sustainability.* Oakland, Calif.: PM Press, 2009.

Kellert, Stephen. "Attitudes and Characteristics of Hunters and Antihunters." *In Transactions of the 43rd North American Wildlife and Natural Resources Conference.* Washington, D.C.: Wildlife Management Institute, 1978.

Kellogg, John Harvey. *Biologic Living: Rules for Right Living.* Battle Creek, Mich.: n.p., 1920.

Kerstetter, Jane E., Anne M. Kenny, and Karl L. Insogna. "Dietary Protein and Skeletal Health: A Review of Recent Human Research." Abstract. *Current Opinion in Lipidology* 22, no. 1 (2011): 16–20. http://journals.lww.com/co-lipidology/pages/articleviewer.aspx?year=2011&issue=02000&article=00005& type=abstract

Kniskern, Megan A., and Carol S. Johnston. "Protein Dietary Reference Intakes May Be Inadequate for Vegetarians If Low Amounts of Animal Protein Are Consumed." *Nutrition* 27, no. 6 (2011): 727–30.

Kummerow, Fred. "Protein: Building Blocks of the Body." *Wise Traditions in Food, Farming and the Healing Arts* (Fall 2011). Weston A. Price Foundation. www.westonaprice.org/vegetarianism-and-plant-foods/protein-building-blocks-of-the-body

Lappé, Frances Moore. *Diet for a Small Planet: Twentieth Anniversary Edition.* New York: Random House Publishing Group, 2011. Kindle edition.

Laurie, W. "Atherosclerosis and Its Cerebral Complications in the South African Bantu." *The Lancet* 271, no. 7014 (1958): 231–32.

Liu, KeShun. *Soybeans: Chemistry, Technology, and Utilization.* New York: Chapman & Hall, 1997.

Madhaven, T. V., and C. Gopalan. "The Effect of Dietary Protein on Carcinogenesis of Aflatoxin." *Archives of Pathology and Laboratory Medicine* 85, no. 2 (1968): 133–37.

Mainigi, K. D., and T. C. Campbell. "Subcellular Distribution and Covalent Binding of Aflatoxins as Functions of Dietary Manipulation." Abstract. *Journal of Toxicology and Environmental Health,* Part A 6, no. 3 (1980): 659–71. PubMed. www.ncbi.nlm.nih.gov/pubmed/7420472

Manninen, Anssi H. "High-Protein Weight Loss Diets and Purported Adverse Effects: Where Is the Evidence?" *Journal of the International Society of Sports Nutrition* 1, no. 1 (2004): 45. www.jissn.com/content/1/1/45

Martin, William F., Lawrence E. Armstrong, and Nancy R. Rodriguez. "Dietary Protein Intake and Renal Function." *Nutrition & Metabolism* 2, no. 25 (2005). BioMed Central. www.nutritionandmetabolism.com/content/pdf/1743-7075-2-25.pdf

Masterjohn, Chris. "On the Trail of the Elusive X-Factor: A Sixty-Two-Year-Old Mystery Finally Solved." *Wise Traditions in Food, Farming and the Healing Arts 8.1* (2007). Weston A. Price Foundation. www.westonaprice.org/fat-soluble-activators/x-factor-is-vitamin-k2

———. "The Curious Case of Campbell's Rats: Does Protein Deficiency Prevent Cancer?" Blog post. Weston A. Price Foundation (September 22, 2010). www.westonaprice.org/blogs/2010/09/22/the-curious-case-of-campbells-rats-does-protein-deficiency-prevent-cancer/

———. "Meat, Organs, Bones, and Skin: Nutrition for Mental Health." Wise Traditions 2012: 13th Annual Conference of the Weston A. Price Foundation. Santa Clara, Calif. (November 2012). Lecture.

———. "The Truth About the China Study." *Cholesterol-and-health.com,* n.d. www.cholesterol-and-health.com/China-Study.html

McGill, H. C., et al. "General Findings of the International Atherosclerosis Project." *Laboratory Investigations* 18, no. 5 (1968): 498–502.

Micha, Renata, Sarah K. Wallace, and Dariush Mozaffarian. "Red and Processed Meat Consumption and Risk of Incident Coronary Heart Disease, Stroke, and Diabetes Mellitus: A Systematic Review and Meta-Analysis." Abstract. *Circulation* 121, no. 21 (2010): 2271–83. http://circ.ahajournals.org/content/121/21/2271.abstract

Michalak, Johannes, Xiao Chi Zhang, and Frank Jacobi. "Vegetarian Diet and Mental Disorders: Results from a Representative Community Survey." *International Journal of Behavioral Nutrition and Physical Activity* 9, no. 67 (2012). www.ijbnpa.org/content/9/1/67

Milton, Katharine. "A Hypothesis to Explain the Role of Meat-Eating in Human Evolution." *Evolutionary Anthropology* 8, no. 1 (1999): 11–21.

Minger, Denise. "'The China Study': A Formal Analysis and Response." *Raw Food SOS.* 2 Aug. 2010. http://rawfoodsos.com/2010/08/06/final-china-study-response-html/

"National Cardiovascular Disease Surveillance." Centers for Disease Control and Prevention, Division for Heart Disease and Stroke Prevention (July 30, 2013). www.cdc.gov/DHDSP/ncvdss/index.htm

National Research Council. *Dietary Reference Intakes for Energy, Carbohydrate, Fiber, Fat, Fatty Acids, Cholesterol, Protein, and Amino Acids (Macronutrients).* Washington, D.C.: The National Academies Press, 2005. www.nap.edu/catalog.php?record_id=10490

———. *Sodium Intake in Populations: Assessment of Evidence.* Washington, D.C.: The National Academies Press, 2013. www.nap.edu/catalog.php?record_id=18311

Nelson, Richard K. *Heart and Blood: Living with Deer in America.* New York: Alfred A. Knopf, 1997.

Ogden, Cynthia, and Margaret Carroll. "Prevalence of Obesity Among Children and Adolescents: United States, Trends 1963–1965 Through 2007–2008." *NCHS Health E-Stat* (2010). Centers for Disease Control and Prevention. www.cdc.gov/nchs/data/hestat/obesity_child_07_08/obesity_child_07_08.htm

The Oiling of America: How the Vegetable Oil Industry Demonized Nutritious Animal Fats and Destroyed the American Food Supply. Derick Moore, director. Derick Moore Productions, 2008. DVD.

Ravnskov, Uffe. *The Cholesterol Myths: Exposing the Fallacy That Cholesterol and Saturated Fat Cause Heart Disease.* Washington, D.C.: NewTrends Publishing, 2000.

———. *Ignore the Awkward!: How the Cholesterol Myths Are Kept Alive.* Charleston, S.C.: CreateSpace, 2010. Kindle edition.

Ross, Julia. *The Mood Cure: The 4-Step Program to Take Charge of Your Emotions—Today.* New York: Penguin Group, 2003. Kindle edition.

Schulsinger, D. A., M. M. Root, and T. C. Campbell. "Effect of Dietary Protein Quality on Development of Aflatoxin B1-Induced Hepatic Preneoplastic Lesions." Abstract. *Journal of the National Cancer Institute* 81, no. 16 (1989): 1241–45. PubMed. www.ncbi.nlm.nih.gov/pubmed/2569044

Schwarz, Richard W. *John Harvey Kellogg, M.D.: Pioneering Health Reformer.* Hagerstown, Md.: Review and Herald Pub. Association, 2006.

Seneff, Stephanie. "Cholesterol, Sulfate, Lactate, and Sunlight: A New Paradigm for Health." Wise Traditions 2011: 12th Annual Conference of the Weston A. Price Foundation. Dallas. (November 2011). Lecture.

———. "Taurine: A Mysterious Molecule with Intriguing Possibilities." Wise Traditions 2012: 13th Annual Conference of the Weston A. Price Foundation. Santa Clara, Calif. (November 12, 2012). Lecture. http://people.csail.mit.edu/seneff/WAPF_Slides_2012/taurine_2012.pdf

Shanahan, Catherine, and Luke Shanahan. *Deep Nutrition: Why Your Genes Need Traditional Food*. Lawai, Hawaii: Big Box, 2009.

Tortora, Gerard J., and Bryan Derrickson. *Introduction to the Human Body: The Essentials of Anatomy and Physiology*, 8th ed. New York: John Wiley & Sons, 2009.

Tudge, Colin. *The Time Before History: 5 Million Years of Human Impact*. New York: Scribner, 1996.

United States Central Intelligence Agency. *The World Factbook*, 2007. www.cia.gov/library/publications/download/download-2007/

Watanabe, F. "Vitamin B12 Sources and Bioavailability." *Experimental Biology and Medicine* 232, no. 10 (2007): 1266–74.

Wrangham, Richard. *Catching Fire: How Cooking Made Us Human*. New York: Basic Books, 2009.

CHAPTER 3: CARBS

Burkitt, Denis Parsons. "Are Our Commonest Diseases Preventable?" *Preventive Medicine* 6, no. 4 (1977): 556–59.

Callaway, Ewen. "Pottery Shards Put a Date on Africa's Dairying." *Nature* (June 20, 2012). www.nature.com/news/pottery-shards-put-a-date-on-africa-s-dairying-1.10863

Carbohydrates in Human Nutrition. Rome: Food and Agriculture Organization of the United Nations, 1997. FAO Food and Nutrition Paper. FAO Corporate Document Repository. www.fao.org/docrep/W8079E/w8079e00.htm

Drago, Sandro, et al. "Gliadin, Zonulin and Gut Permeability: Effect on Celiac and Non-celiac Intestinal Mucosa and Intestinal Cell Lines." Abstract. *Scandinavian Journal of Gastroenterology* 41, no. 4 (2006): 408–19. PubMed. www.ncbi.nlm.nih.gov/pubmed/16635908

"The Facts about Real Raw Milk." *A Campaign for Real Milk* (February 28, 2013). www.realmilk.com

Fasano, Alessio. "Intestinal Permeability and Its Regulation by Zonulin: Diagnostic and Therapeutic Implications." *Clinical Gastroenterology and Hepatology* 10, no. 10 (2012): 1096–1100.

Fasano, Alessio. "Zonulin and Its Regulation of Intestinal Barrier Function: The Biological Door to Inflammation, Autoimmunity, and Cancer." *Physiological Reviews* 91, no.1 (2011): 151–75. http://physrev.physiology.org/content/91/1/151.long

———. "Zonulin, Regulation of Tight Junctions, and Autoimmune Diseases." *Annals of the New York Academy of Sciences* 1258 (2012): 25–33.

"Grain Harvest Sets Record, But Supplies Still Tight." *Worldwatch Institute,* n.d.

Harcombe, Zoë. *The Obesity Epidemic: What Caused It? How Can We Stop It?* U.K.: Columbus Digital Services Ltd, 2010. Kindle edition.

Ikerd, John E. *Crisis and Opportunity: Sustainability in American Agriculture.* Lincoln: University of Nebraska Press, 2008. Our Sustainable Future. Kindle edition.

Jackson, Jessica R. "Neurologic and Psychiatric Manifestations of Celiac Disease and Gluten Sensitivity." *Psychiatric Quarterly* 83, no. 1 (2012): 91–102.

Maize in Human Nutrition. *Rome: Food and Agriculture Organization of the United Nations,* 1992. FAO Corporate Document Repository. www.fao.org/docrep/t0395e/T0395E00.htm

Mason, John. *Sustainable Agriculture.* Collingwood, Victoria, Australia: Landlinks Press, 2003. Kindle edition.

McFerron, Whitney. "Livestock Eat More Wheat as Cheapest Corn Alternative Since 1996." *Bloomberg.com.* (June 14, 2011). www.bloomberg.com/news/2011-06-14/livestock-eat-more-wheat-as-cheapest-corn-alternative-since-1996.html

Nachbar, Martin S., and Joel D. Oppenheim. "Lectins in the United States Diet: A Survey of Lectins in Commonly Consumed Foods and a Review of the Literature." *American Journal of Clinical Nutrition* 33, no. 11 (1980): 2338–45. http://ajcn.nutrition.org/content/33/11/2338.full.pdf

Nestle, Marion. *Food Politics: How the Food Industry Influences Nutrition and Health.* Berkeley: University of California Press, 2002.

Park, Y., et al. "Dietary Fiber Intake and Risk of Colorectal Cancer: A Pooled Analysis of Prospective Cohort Studies." *Journal of the American Medical Association* 294, no. 22 (2005): 2849–57.

Price, Weston A. *Nutrition and Physical Degeneration: A Comparison of Primitive and Modern Diets and Their Effects*, 8th ed. La Mesa, Calif.: Price-Pottenger Nutrition Foundation, 2008.

Reddy, N. Rukma, and Shridhar K. Sathe, eds. *Food Phytates.* Boca Raton, Fla.: CRC Press, 2002.

Rich, Deborah K. "The Case Against Synthetic Fertilizers: Industrial Process Opens Door to Many Environmental Risks." *San Francisco Chronicle* (January 14, 2006). *SF Gate.* www.sfgate.com/homeandgarden/article/The-case-against-synthetic-fertilizers-2506802.php

Schmid, Ronald F. *The Untold Story of Milk: The History, Politics and Science of Nature's Perfect Food: Raw Milk from Pasture-Fed Cows.* Washington, D.C.: NewTrends Publishing, Inc., 2009.

Shanahan, Catherine, and Luke Shanahan. *Deep Nutrition: Why Your Genes Need Traditional Food.* Lawai, Hawaii: Big Box, 2009.

Story, Jon A., and David Kritchevsky. "Denis Parsons Burkitt (1911–1993)." *Journal of Nutrition* 124 (1994): 1551–54. http://jn.nutrition.org/content/124/9/1551.full.pdf

Sweets, Laura E., and J. Allen Wrather. "Aflatoxin in Corn." University of Missouri Fisher Delta Research Center, Agriculture Experiment Station. University of Missouri College of Agriculture, Food, and Natural Resources (March 2009). http://aes.missouri.edu/delta/croppest/aflacorn.stm

Taubes, Gary. *Good Calories, Bad Calories: Challenging the Conventional Wisdom on Diet, Weight Control, and Disease.* New York: Alfred A. Knopf, 2007.

Tudge, Colin. *The Time Before History: 5 Million Years of Human Impact.* New York: Scribner, 1996.

United States Department of Agriculture. *ChooseMyPlate.gov.* http://choosemyplate.gov.

United States Department of Agriculture and Department of Health and Human Services. *Dietary Guidelines for Americans 2010, 7th ed. Washington,* D.C.: U.S. Government Printing Office, 2010. *Health.gov.* www.health.gov/dietaryguidelines/dga2010/DietaryGuidelines2010.pdf

United States Food and Drug Administration. "Arsenic and Rice in Rice Products" (September 12, 2013). www.fda.gov/Food/FoodborneIllness Contaminants/Metals/ucm319870.htm

CHAPTER 4: NUTRIENTS

Amizuka, N., M. Li, Y. Guo, et al. "Biological Effects of Vitamin K2 on Bone Quality." Abstract. *Clinical Calcium* 19, no. 12 (2009): 1788–96. PubMed. www.ncbi.nlm.nih.gov/pubmed/19949270

Armstrong, B. K., and A. Kricker. "Skin Cancer." Abstract. *Dermatologic Clinics 13*, no. 3 (1995): 583–94. PubMed. www.ncbi.nlm.nih.gov/pubmed/7554506

Bayer, Ronald, David Merritt Johns, and Sandro Galea. "Salt and Public Health: Contested Science and the Challenge of Evidence-Based Decision Making." *Health Affairs* 31, no. 12 (2012): 2738–46.

Bitterman, Mark. *Salted: A Manifesto on the World's Most Essential Mineral, with Recipes.* Berkeley, Calif.: Ten Speed Press, 2010. Kindle edition.

Bosch, J., et al. "n-3 Fatty Acids and Cardiovascular Outcomes in Patients with Dysglycemia." *New England Journal of Medicine* 367, no. 4 (2012): 309–18. www.nejm.org/doi/full/10.1056/NEJMoa1203859

Brenner, Michaela, and Vincent J. Hearing. "The Protective Role of Melanin against UV Damage in Human Skin." *Photochemistry and Photobiology* 84, no. 3 (2008): 539–49. PubMed Central. www.ncbi.nlm.nih.gov/pmc/articles/PMC2671032/

Buchholz, Andrea C., and Dale A. Schoeller. "Is a Calorie a Calorie?" *American Journal of Clinical Nutrition* 79, no. 5 (2004): 899S–906S. http://ajcn.nutrition.org/content/79/5/899S.long

Coll, Anthony P., I. Sadaf Farooqi, and Stephen O'Rahilly. "The Hormonal Control of Food Intake." *Cell* 129, no. 2 (2007): 251–62. PubMed Central. www.ncbi.nlm.nih.gov/pmc/articles/PMC2202913/

Dam, Henrik. "The Discovery of Vitamin K, Its Biological Functions and Therapeutical Application." Nobel Lecture (December 12, 1946). *Nobelprize.org*. Nobel Foundation. www.nobelprize.org/nobel_prizes/medicine/laureates/1943/dam-lecture.pdf

Davis, Brenda C., and Penny M. Kris-Etherton. "Achieving Optimal Essential Fatty Acid Status in Vegetarians: Current Knowledge and Practical Implications." *American Journal of Clinical Nutrition* 78, no. 3 (2003): 640S–646S. http://ajcn.nutrition.org/content/78/3/640S.long

Dean, Carolyn. *The Magnesium Miracle*. New York: Random House, 2007. Kindle edition.

"The Discovery of Insulin." *Nobelprize.org*. Nobel Media AB (2013). www.nobelprize.org/educational/medicine/insulin/discovery-insulin.html

Dunne, L. J. *Nutrition Almanac*, 3rd ed. New York: McGraw-Hill Publishing Company, 1990. Via Fallon, Sally, and Mary G. Enig. "Vitamin A Saga." Weston A. Price Foundation (March 30, 2002). www.westonaprice.org/fat-soluble-activators/vitamin-a-saga

Enig, Mary G. *Know Your Fats: The Complete Primer for Understanding the Nutrition of Fats, Oils, and Cholesterol*. Silver Spring, Md.: Bethesda Press, 2000.

Erlich, Steven D. "Vitamin A (Retinol)." University of Maryland Medical Center (June 21, 2013). http://umm.edu/health/medical/altmed/supplement/vitamin-a-retinol

"Europe's Better Sunscreens." *EWG's 2013 Guide to Sunscreens*. Environmental Working Group, n.d. www.ewg.org/2013sunscreen/europes-better-sunscreens/

Factory Farm Nation: How America Turned Its Livestock Farms into Factories. Report. Food & Water Watch (November 2010). www.factoryfarmmap.org/wp-content/uploads/2010/11/FactoryFarmNation-web.pdf

"FDA Fails Consumers." *EWG's 2013 Guide to Sunscreen*. Environmental Working Group, n.d. www.ewg.org/2013sunscreen/fda-fails-consumers/

Feinman, Richard D., and Eugene J. Fine. "Thermodynamics and Metabolic Advantage of Weight Loss Diets." *Metabolic Syndrome and Related Disorders* 1, no. 3 (2003): 209–19.

Foley, T. P., Jr. "The Relationship between Autoimmune Thyroid Disease and Iodine Intake: A Review." Abstract. *Endokrynologia Polska* 43, Supplement 1 (1992): 53–69. PubMed. www.ncbi.nlm.nih.gov/pubmed/1345585

Gloster, H. M., Jr., and D. G. Brodland. "The Epidemiology of Skin Cancer." Abstract. *Dermatologic Surgery* 22, no. 3 (1996): 217–26. PubMed. www.ncbi. nlm.nih.gov/pubmed/8599733

Godar, Dianne E., Robert J. Landry, and Anne D. Lucas. "Increased UVA Exposures and Decreased Cutaneous Vitamin D3 Levels May Be Responsible for the Increasing Incidence of Melanoma." Abstract. *Medical Hypotheses* 72, no. 4 (2009): 434–43. www.medical-hypotheses.com/article/S0306-9877(08)00599-9/ abstract

Graudal, Niels, and Gesche Jürgens. "Letter: The Sodium Phantom." BMJ 343 (2011). www.bmj.com/content/343/bmj.d6119

Guyenet, Stephan. "Vitamin K2 and Cranial Development." *Whole Health Source: Nutrition and Health Science* (January 27, 2009). http://wholehealth-source.blogspot.com/2009/01/vitamin-k2-and-cranial-development.html

———. "Whole Health Source: Reversing Tooth Decay." *Whole Health Source: Nutrition and Health Science* (April 1, 2009). http://wholehealthsource. blogspot.com/2009/03/reversing-tooth-decay.html

———. "Malocclusion: Disease of Civilization, Part V." *Whole Health Source: Nutrition and Health Science* (November 10, 2009). http://wholehealthsource. blogspot.com/2009/11/malocclusion-disease-of-civilization.html

———. "Dr. Mellanby's Tooth Decay Reversal Diet." *Whole Health Source: Nutrition and Health Science* (December 11, 2010). http://wholehealthsource. blogspot.com/2010/12/dr-mellanbys-tooth-decay-reversal-diet.html

Hall, H., D. Miller, J. Rogers, and B. Bewerse. "Update on the Incidence and Mortality from Melanoma in the United States." Abstract. *Journal of the American Academy of Dermatology* 40, no. 1 (1999): 35–42. PubMed. www.ncbi. nlm.nih.gov/pubmed/9922010

Harcombe, Zoë. *The Obesity Epidemic: What Caused It? How Can We Stop It?* UK: Columbus Digital Services Ltd., 2010. Kindle edition.

Hargrove, James L. "History of the Calorie in Nutrition." *Journal of Nutrition* 136, no. 12 (2006): 2957–61. http://nutrition.highwire.org/content/136/12/2957. full

"Health Conditions." Vitamin D Council, n.d. www.vitamindcouncil.org/ health-conditions/

Herper, Matthew. "Fish Oil or Snake Oil? Study Questions Omega-3 Benefits." *Forbes.* (June 11, 2012). www.forbes.com/sites/matthewherper/2012/06/11/ fish-oil-or-snake-oil-study-questions-omega-3-benefits/

Higdon, Jane, and Victoria Drake. *An Evidence-Based Approach to Vitamins and Minerals: Health Benefits and Intake Recommendations.* Stuttgart, Germany: Thieme Medical Publishers, 2011. Kindle edition.

Holick, Michael F. *The Vitamin D Solution: A 3-Step Strategy to Cure Our Most Common Health Problems.* New York: Hudson Street Press, 2010.

Holt, Douglas B. "Got Milk?" Advertising Educational Foundation (2002). www.aef.com/on_campus/classroom/case_histories/3000

Horrocks, Lloyd A., and Young K. Leo. "Health Benefits of Docosahexaenoic Acid (DHA)." *Pharmacological Research* 40, no. 3 (1999): 211–25.

Khalsa, Soram. *The Vitamin D Revolution: How the Power of This Amazing Vitamin Can Change Your Life*. Carlsbad, Calif.: Hay House, 2009. Kindle edition.

Kurlansky, Mark. *Salt: A World History*. New York: Penguin, 2003. Kindle edition.

Lange, J. R., B. E. Palis, D. C. Chang, et al. "Melanoma in Children and Teenagers: An Analysis of Patients From the National Cancer Data Base." *Journal of Clinical Oncology* 25, no. 11 (2007): 1363–68.

Lassek, William D., and Steven J. C. Gaulin. *Why Women Need Fat: How "Healthy" Food Makes Us Gain Excess Weight and the Surprising Solution to Losing It Forever*. New York: Hudson Street Press, 2012. Kindle edition.

Leaf, Alexander. "Historical Overview of n-3 Fatty Acids and Coronary Heart Disease." *American Journal of Clinical Nutrition* 87, Supplement (2008): 1978S–1980S. http://ajcn.nutrition.org/content/87/6/1978S.full.pdf

Li, Min-Dian. "Leptin and Beyond: An Odyssey to the Central Control of Body Weight." *Yale Journal of Biology and Medicine* 84, no. 1 (2011): 1–7. PubMed Central. www.ncbi.nlm.nih.gov/pmc/articles/PMC3064240/

Lustig, Robert H. *Fat Chance: Beating the Odds Against Sugar, Processed Food, Obesity, and Disease*. New York: Hudson Street, 2012. Kindle edition.

Marshall, Trevor G. "Vitamin D Discovery Outpaces FDA Decision Making." Abstract. *BioEssays* 30, no. 2 (2008): 173–82. Wiley Online Library (January 15, 2008). http://onlinelibrary.wiley.com/doi/10.1002/bies.20708/abstract

Masella, Roberta, and Giuseppe Mazza, eds. *Glutathione and Sulfur Amino Acids in Human Health and Disease*. Hoboken, N.J.: John Wiley & Sons, 2009.

Masterjohn, Chris. "Vitamin A on Trial: Does Vitamin A Cause Osteoporosis?" *Wise Traditions in Food, Farming and the Healing Arts* 7, no. 1 (2005/2006). Weston A. Price Foundation. www.westonaprice.org/fat-soluble-activators/vitamin-a-on-trial

———. "How Essential Are the Essential Fatty Acids? The PUFA Report Part 1: A Critical Review of the Requirement for Polyunsaturated Fatty Acids." *Cholesterol-And-Health.Com Special Reports* 1, no. 2 (2008). www.cholesterol-and-health.com/PUFA-Special-Report.html.

———. "On the Trail of the Elusive X-Factor: A Sixty-Two-Year-Old Mystery Finally Solved." *Wise Traditions in Food, Farming and the Healing Arts* 8, no. 1 (2007). Weston A. Price Foundation. www.westonaprice.org/fat-soluble-activators/x-factor-is-vitamin-k2

McGee, Harold. *On Food and Cooking: The Science and Lore of the Kitchen*. New York: Scribner, 2004. Kindle edition.

Moss, Michael. *Salt, Sugar, Fat: How the Food Giants Hooked Us*. New York: Random House, 2013. Kindle edition.

National Research Council. *Sodium Intake in Populations: Assessment of Evidence*. Washington, D.C.: The National Academies Press, 2013. www.nap.edu/catalog.php?record_id=18311

Paltrow, Gwyneth. "Vitamin D." *goop.com* (June 16, 2010). http://goop.com/journal/do/88/vitamin-d

Pellett, Peter L. "Commentary: The R.D.A. Controversy Revisited." *Ecology of Food and Nutrition* 21, no. 4 (1988): 315–20. www.tandfonline.com/doi/abs/10.1080/03670244.1988.9991045

Plourde, Elizabeth. *Sunscreens—Biohazard: Treat as Hazardous Waste*. Irvine, Calif.: New Voice Publications, 2012. Kindle edition.

"Process." *The Production of Fish Meal and Oil*. Rome: Food and Agriculture Organization of the United Nations, 1986. FAO Fisheries Technical Paper. FAO Corporate Document Repository. www.fao.org/docrep/003/x6899e/x6899e04.htm

Rajakumar, Kumaravel. "Vitamin D, Cod-Liver Oil, Sunlight, and Rickets: A Historical Perspective." *Pediatrics* 112, no. 2 (2003): E132–35. http://pediatrics.aappublications.org/content/112/2/e132.full.h

Rhéaume-Bleue, Kate. *Vitamin K$_2$ and the Calcium Paradox: How a Little-Known Vitamin Could Save Your Life,* reprint ed. Mississauga, Ont.: HarperCollins Canada, 2012. Kindle edition.

Richards, Byron J., and Mary Guignon Richards. *Mastering Leptin: Your Guide to Permanent Weight Loss and Optimum Health*. Minneapolis: Wellness Resources, 2009. Kindle edition.

Rivers, Jason K. "Is There More than One Road to Melanoma?" *The Lancet* 363, no. 9410 (2004): 728–30. www.thelancet.com/journals/lancet/article/PIIS0140-6736%2804%2915649-3/fulltext

Rothman, Kenneth J., Lynn L. Moore, Martha R. Singer, et al. "Teratogenicity of High Vitamin A Intake." *New England Journal of Medicine* 333 (1995): 1369–73. www.nejm.org/doi/full/10.1056/NEJM199511233332101

Schmid, Ronald F. *The Untold Story of Milk: The History, Politics and Science of Nature's Perfect Food: Raw Milk from Pasture-fed Cows*. Washington, D.C.: NewTrends Pub., 2009.

Schneider, Andrew. "Study: Many Sunscreens May Be Accelerating Cancer." *AOL News*. (May 24, 2010). www.aolnews.com/2010/05/24/study-many-sunscreens-may-be-accelerating-cancer/

Schwartz, M. W. "Adiposity Signaling and Biological Defense against Weight Gain: Absence of Protection or Central Hormone Resistance?" *Journal of Clinical Endocrinology and Metabolism* 89, no. 12 (2004): 5889–97. http://jcem.endojournals.org/content/89/12/5889.long

Self Nutrition Data. Self. http://nutritiondata.self.com

Seneff, Stephanie. "Cholesterol, Sulfur, Lactate, and Sunlight: A New Paradigm for Health." MIT Computer Science and Artificial Intelligence Laboratory, n.d. http://people.csail.mit.edu/seneff/

"Shaking the Salt Habit." American Heart Association (April 22, 2013). www. heart.org/HEARTORG/Conditions/HighBloodPressure/Prevention TreatmentofHighBloodPressure/Shaking-the-Salt-Habit_UCM_303241_ Article.jsp

Shanahan, Catherine, and Luke Shanahan. *Deep Nutrition: Why Your Genes Need Traditional Food*. Lawai, Hawaii: Big Box, 2009.

"Skin Cancer on the Rise." *EWG's 2013 Guide to Sunscreens*. Environmental Working Group. www.ewg.org/2013sunscreen/skin-cancer-on-the-rise/

Specker, Bonny L. "Should There Be a Dietary Guideline for Calcium Intake? No." *American Journal of Clinical Nutrition* 71, no. 3 (2000): 661–64. http://ajcn. nutrition.org/content/71/3/661.full

Stolarz-Skrzypek, Katarzyna, et al. "Fatal and Nonfatal Outcomes, Incidence of Hypertension, and Blood Pressure Changes in Relation to Urinary Sodium Excretion." *Journal of the American Medical Association* 305, no. 17 (2011): 1777–85. http://jama.jamanetwork.com/article.aspx?articleid=899663

"Sunscreen Manufacturing in the US: Market Research Report." Sample. *IBISWorld* (November 2012). www.ibisworld.com/industry/sunscreen-manufacturing.html

Swanson, Danielle, Robert Block, and Shaker A. Mousa. "Omega-3 Fatty Acids EPA and DHA: Health Benefits Throughout Life." *Advances in Nutrition* 3 (2012): 1–7. http://advances.nutrition.org/content/3/1/1.full

Wheeler, Sally M., G. H. Fleet, and R. J. Ashley. "Effect of Processing upon Concentration and Distribution of Natural and Lodophor-Derived Iodine in Milk." *Journal of Dairy Science* 66, no. 2 (1983): 187–95.

Wolf, George. "The Discovery of Vitamin D: The Contribution of Adolf Windaus." *Journal of Nutrition* 134, no. 6 (2004): 1299–1302. http://jn.nutrition. org/content/134/6/1299.full

Zofková, I., and R. L. Kancheva. "The Relationship between Magnesium and Calciotropic Hormones." *Magnesium Research* 8, no. 1 (1995): 77–84.

index